CLIMBING BACK:
A JOURNEY WITH CANCER

22 Feb 99

For Jean Wigham,

   With great respect,
admiration, and hopes
that whatever challenges
life presents, you'll
find strength from
within and from those
who know a love
you.

       Best wishe
      Mah Ge

CLIMBING BACK:
A JOURNEY WITH CANCER

MARK H. GERNER

Kroshka Books
Commack, New York

Editorial Production: Susan Boriotti
Office Manager: Annette Hellinger
Graphics: Frank Grucci and John T'Lustachowski
Information Editor: Tatiana Shohov
Book Production: Donna Dennis, Patrick Davin, Christine Mathosian, Tammy Sauter and Diane Sharp
Circulation: Maryanne Schmidt
Marketing/Sales: Cathy DeGregory

Library of Congress Cataloging-in-Publication Data

Gerner, Mark.
      Climbing Back: A Journey With Cancer/ by Mark Gerner.
              p.   cm.
      ISBN 1-56072-512-5
        1. Gerner, Mark--Health. 2. Testis--Cancer--Patients--Biography. I. Title
RC280.T4G476   1998   97-41658
362.1'9699463—dc21   CIP
[B]

Printed in the United States of America

CONTENTS

1 Up and Down 1
2 The Old Life: The Fighter 5
3 Moments 43
4 A New Kind of Fight 67
5 Numb Fingers and Long Falls 85
6 West and East 115
7 "Paint my House" 133
8 Which Way? 157
9 Flows and Steps 169
  Bibliography 179

First and foremost, this book is dedicated to the love of my life, my wife Debra. Only she will know...

It is also for my two sons, Sean and Jeffrey, whose struggles were as great as mine, and who each became my heroes.

It is for Elliott Gruner, Marc Guthartz, Bob Miller, Roger Spiller and Anita McMiller.

It is for the doctors and the nurses, many now nameless, who constantly toil to fight our enduring demons. It is especially for John Vaccarro and for Bill Fox, soldiers like few others.

Finally, it is for Barbara Bachmeier, who offered friendship and encouragement, while she found those places...

1 UP AND DOWN

The world spun above me. All strength in hands, feet, and limbs was spent. Each muscle and tendon told my brain that my body must stop movement and not climb. Below, the closest ledge was a very distant eighty feet and a world away. Above, there was no sign of a secure ledge. My partner managed my lifeline from a place he reached by a different route, leaving me alone with the moves to the top. The smooth rock face did not hold many cracks or changes on its surface. The route would emerge from whatever I could design. My left hand found a way to stretch tired tendons as three fingers could hold a small well while the outside edge of my right foot found a line on the wall. Locking my hip and leg, my right side moved against the roof of the overhang. To my great surprise, it held long enough for my right hand to move higher.

"It isn't possible to fall," I told myself. But at the same moment, my left hand slipped away. Again, the ledge and I hung out over the valley floor.

The autumn day had been crisp and clear, perfect for our climb in the Shawangunk Mountains overlooking Spring Valley, New York. But now the "Gunks" reflected the late October afternoon sunlight. The air turned cold, and threatened to further exhaust already tired muscles. Noises from the valley floor floated up and became audible as children's words and laughter, sounds of Sunday afternoon play. Instead of playing with my two children, I was trying to figure out this puzzle of a climb. Though it was quite improbable that I would fall, my performance over the last hour suggested that I was beyond my level of skill. My solution was not within my limbs; it would have to come from elsewhere.

The pain in each joint of every finger now turned to numbness. The fatigue in my forearms told me my that my technique needed improvement. My legs and feet should have been taking on more weight than my hands and arms. But this was no time for self-criticism. "I'll work on the skill," I told myself. Then I added, quietly talking to myself out loud, "Do this climb. Climb this face. Forget how you would like it to be, take it as it is." The tingling turned sharp. Needles of pain were all over my hands and arms. Then all feeling was gone.

I lay back on the rope, put both feet together into a crack, and breathed deeply. I closed my eyes and slowly awaited some relaxation. I thought of a dynamic move, a way to move feet, arms, and torso at once so as to extend my reach and find the way to the exposed but fast holds that were within sight. Crouching to the left to gather momentum, I thrust my right arm and gave my weight to the new hold. I found my rhythm by rotating hips, crossing my hands over each other onto the surface of the overhanging ledge, while edging alternating feet on the rock face in front of me. I found my balance points, got my weight up, and I began to move. The hundreds of feet of air below no longer meant anything. For the briefest of moments, I gave myself to the rock.

The first hour of effort produced only twelve feet of height, but now I climbed the hundred feet to the top of the pitch in minutes. I stood looking out over the valley, completely spent; blood pumping through chest and arms and ears, and I consumed the view. I did not seriously explore the art of rock climbing until I was thirty-seven years old. Until after it was over.

On the drive home I navigated my way back through the town of New Paltz and the surrounding hills that inspired the Legend of Sleepy Hollow. I soaked in the colors of trees now awash in reds and golds in the fast fading sunlight. From the upper Hudson Valley, I made my way to West Point, the most recent of our many homes. I focused on this remarkable day, nothing more. Alive, in touch with all my senses in ways so strong there was a sensual character to them, I was in my own moment.

I was suddenly jerked back to other feelings. The numbness in my hands and fingers, just minutes ago a part of my soulful climb, now summoned me to a not so distant scene of the past, a time and place of cancer and chemotherapy. I surrendered to the rock, and I climbed it. But I puzzled over my surrender to cancer. My tingling fingertips brought back the ordeal.

My story begins.

2 THE OLD LIFE: THE FIGHTER

My images of cancer intersect with times that reside both within and at the margins of the long battle. The disease engaged me on its own terms, creating illusions with many masks. While I suffered the effects, it played with me. It would take years for me to learn to detect the camouflaged invader's methods, and only through work, thought and spiritual reckoning did I come to understand how I fought the battle.

There was a great mixing of we three: cancer, time, and me. We came together in a kind of dance moving to beats and rhythms that changed over time. We mixed new combinations of steps, sometimes choreographed and predictable, but mostly random and chaotic. At times, the steps ran smoothly along well-designed tracks, perfect in geometric form. They showed great beauty, these moves, even if they came from mysterious and undiscovered sources. At other times, the steps darted with crazy speed and direction, crashing into invisible but solid boundaries that defined my life's limits. Hours flow into weeks and then years. When pain was in the spotlight, my dance partners departed with haste, leaving me alone with my wife and children. When the light found me in healthy times, the disease crouched and hid in the shadows, as if to remind that it can still claim my time.

At its core, cancer is a story, and like most human stories, it rarely ends as it begins. My images move swiftly at first, darting with enthusiasm and intensity, in loud young voices filled with the excitement and the hormones of youth as they negotiate city streets and base lines and grid lines in city parks. They take the base paths faster with each year's added strength and improved muscle memory while I learn to play in the small worlds of green that dot the city neighborhoods. As the years expand, I find my way west, exploring the unknown peaks and ridges that introduce new perspectives, so different from what was known before, until finally they settle in high places that look down upon clouds.

My intimate dance with disease began in a place I had visited before. A day quite apart from my climb in the beautiful "Gunks" floated in front of my mind's eye. It was two and a half years earlier, February 1987. It was typically Pacific Northwest. Cold, dark, and wet, there was the kind of chill that reached into your neck and back and did not let go. I had some small tasks to complete before leaving Fort Lewis for our home in Spanaway, a part of Tacoma, Washington, the most important of which was to begin a routine physical examination. My upcoming thirty-fifth birthday triggered the date. Healthy and fit, I thought nothing of it; the only reason for this appointment was the fulfillment of a military requirement.

The Physicians Assistant had a familiar face. I met him on a recent training exercise, and I liked him.

"Hello, Major. Come in and sit down. I know you're in a hurry, so I'll cover the questions on the form with you, then do some simple checks, and we're done. Take these lab slips for blood tests next week." Then he added, "Sir, I don't see your medical record here. Did you ever process in to the clinic?"

"No, Chief, I've been here since June, but I just never got around to it. Sorry."

"That's OK, I'll do it now. Where was your last duty station, sir?"

"Leavenworth." The place is so widely known within the Army that it is almost a code. Sharing the Kansas town with the prison is the Army's Command and General Staff College, practically required attendance for officers in the grade of major. After the year of school, I was assigned to Fort Lewis as the logistics officer for the first brigade of the Army's 9th Infantry Division in the summer of 1986.

"Have you been stationed here before, Major?" he said as he guided the stethoscope and listened to my breathing. Then he moved to examine lymph nodes under my arms and in my neck.

"Yes. I started out here as a second lieutenant. Got here in 1974 and stayed until '79; I spent the entire time with the Third of the Thirty-Ninth Infantry. I stayed in the same battalion for five years and went from platoon leader to company commander."

"That was about the time Schwarzkopf was the brigade commander, wasn't it?" He referred to Lieutenant General H. Norman Schwarzkopf, who at this time commanded the Army's First Corps at Fort Lewis. Later, he was promoted to four star general and command all forces in the Persian Gulf during operations Desert Shield and Desert Storm. Long before his name was a household word, he was a memorable character to many who served with him.

"I was a company commander in his brigade."

"Well, I hope you enjoy your tour here. I'm leaving soon. I grew up around here and I love it. Many people can't stand the rain, but there's a lot to enjoy here." Then he changed the subject. "How are you feeling?"

"I'm fine, Doc. No problems. My running is good. Faster than I've been in a long time. I feel very good." I was as captured as anyone back then that if I could run well then I could not possibly be sick.

I was about to leave when he caught himself. "Oh, I need to do one more check. Would you take off your underwear and lay back on the table? I have to palpate your testicles."

We continued the small talk; salmon fishing, where to go for steelhead on the Nisqually River, the Mariners. Then his expression changed and speaking in a professional tone he asked, "Have you ever done a self examination on your testicles?"

A cold spot paralyzed the small of my back. I had no idea what he meant.

"Self examination for what?" I said, puzzled.

"Why, for testicular cancer," he said in a manner that suggested everyone knew about the disease and how to check for it.

I had not heard of testicular cancer, not in such specific terms.

When was I supposed to have found this? What was I supposed to do?

The dark day's chill sunk deep into my spine, spreading paralysis to chest, lungs, arms, face, and my mind. My vague sense of ignorance was displaced by a sharp image of fear.

"Sir, I may be wrong, but that knot on your testicle looks like a tumor. I'll call Doctor Fox at the urology clinic. He needs to see you. I'm not able to give you a real diagnosis. I just know that a knot like that is a sign, and you need to see a urologist. Get dressed, please, and I'll call him.

I was watching myself in a slow motion movie. I could hear Fox's voice through the phone. He sounded hurried and

bothered, yet anxious to see me right away. He told the
Physician's Assistant to send me "now, right now." My feet felt
planted in cement and I went a little faint as I rose. "Why
couldn't this wait until Monday?" I asked only myself.

I promised the "PA" that I would come back and tell him
how I was, but I never did. In the ten minutes that ticked off the
clock as I drove to Madigan Army Medical Center, I told myself
that cancer could not happen to me, that the examination had to
be wrong. The lump was something else; the urologist would
know better, and all of this would be settled in an hour. But I
also knew that I had to face this, whatever it was, and I had to so
clearly and unemotionally. There would be no room for denial.

*Just go do what he said. Go to this Fox and let him do
his thing.*

The mist had turned to a cold rain, but one of those famously
unpredictable warm Chinook winds blew over me as I walked
the few blocks to the clinic. Scents of rain and pine mixed and
rolled together like lovers. I breathed deeply, drinking in the air,
considering how this place suited me. I breathed as if the wind
were an omen. A bothersome thought came from nowhere.
...Enjoy this now, while you still can. But quickly threw the
frightening thought aside, and walked in to meet the urologist.

The urology clinic was a very busy place. People of all ages
were coming and going, some with bags of medicine. One older
man carefully holding his new surgically attached bag with old,
leathery hands. He gives me a quick, knowing look. A young
boy, four or five, sitting quietly, trying to sleep. His mother
engulfs him in her clearly tired arms. I enter her field of view,
but she doesn't see me or anyone else as she gently puts a tissue
first to his large brown eyes, then to her own very red ones. She
has the look of someone seeing another time. The receptionist,

an attractive lady in her fifties changed her expressions rapidly and skillfully with each name she called. She offered a little something personal to the six people in line ahead of me, looking each one in the eye and speaking softly with her strong but gentle German accent. She seems a quiet port in this storm of confused and anxious people. Her face is filled with conflict. Her eyes and voice are each strong and business-like while describing some pills to a man in his seventies. Then she smiles warmly as she bids him farewell and calls him by name. Between patients, she nervously checks her watch. A dinner date with her husband? Cleaning to pick up before the weekend? Or maybe a sick son or grandson to visit? Maybe she is simply worn out after a week of this hectic pace. Maybe.

When she saw my name tape on my uniform pocket, she seemed to light up.

"Oh, Major Gerner! We've been waiting for you. Please, go in and see Doctor Fox right now." Her eyes locked on mine. They seemed to say that I should not worry, that people here would take care of me. But a trace of conflict was also there as they hinted that the doctor had already given her instructions about me. It was a bit of an eerie feeling. I thanked her and went into to meet the doctor.

He was handsome, young, and obviously very bright. He smiled genuinely and shook my hand with warmth and a little sympathy as he simply said, "Hello, I am Bill Fox. Let's see what's going on here."

I did not even need to lie down. I simply dropped my pants and underwear. He looked at the knot for about thirty seconds and said, "Well, that's got to come out. We'll get you into surgery tonight. You can put your pants on now."

That's it? Come over for a checkup and go in for surgery. Great weekend. I wonder who else is going to tell

me to take my trousers up and down before today is one.
Isn't he going to explain any of this?

He was a Special Forces officer and his office walls were
plastered with tributes to his personal adventures. Africa with
some remote aid station, parachute drops, some Mobile Army
Surgical Hospital (MASH) team on some dusty airstrip
somewhere. Thailand? The Philippines? I found myself hoping I
was not a new adventure. I got up the nerve to ask, "Are you sure
about this? Shouldn't we get another opinion before you just cut
this out?"

I also had to get up the courage to tell him the embarrassing
truth. I noticed the knot on my testicle four months earlier, but I
never recognized it as anything other than some innocent
infection. I was also uneasy about a distant childhood memory.
When I was ten years old, my neighborhood friends' mother
would scream out to him, "Put on clean underwear. You never
know if you'll be in an accident and they'll take you to the
hospital and then everyone will see you have dirty underwear.
Everybody will think I'm a terrible mother, letting you go out
like that."

Fox interrupted my escape into childhood with an offer of a
second opinion. A visiting urologist from Seattle, a woman
doctor who was part of the teaching program, offered to examine
me. My brief hope that a second opinion would save the
weekend and maybe the testicle was dashed on the rocks of
reality. Once again, down came the pants, and now two doctors
viewed my testicles as well as my friend's mother's prophetic
fear: dirty underwear.

"As soon as I leave here they are going to start talking about
the major who wears dirty underwear," I recall telling myself.
My childhood memory may have had a practical side. A
childhood condition frequently associated with testicular cancer

later in life is cryterchidism, when the testicles do not naturally descend into the scrotum to occupy the proper place. I fit that pattern. Mine did not descend until about age eight. Though not proven in a statistical sense, there is enough anecdotal evidence of this connection to at least warn men who may have had this condition to be extra cautious with self-examination. I knew none of this back then.

They both told me, almost in harmony, "You can put your pants on now." (I was starting to keep score. It was now four times that I received this command today.) I asked them, "Why do you have to remove the testicle? Can't you just take out the growth?"

They looked at each other and their eyes agreed that the woman doctor should deliver the answer.

"That isn't how these tumors work," she began. "It's not a pimple or an infection. We can tell by its size, shape and color that it is a tumor. The only way to remove it to take out the entire testicle. It has to come out or the disease will spread. Your other testicle should continue to function normally."

Suddenly the old joke about "Don't worry about losing your arm, leg, or whatever, you have another one, was not so funny.

While I listened to her, I sensed that Doctor Fox was watching me carefully. I was not sure what to make of Bill Fox. Was he "knife happy" and just wanted more cancer patients? But as I watched him, I knew I would surrender to his judgment and accept the surgery.

I walked slowly to the hospital's distant admissions office. "How are you going to manage this?" I asked out loud. "You have all of these other things to do. How much time will this take? Am I in to this for the weekend or for years? No one is mentioning that part of it yet."

The building was a labyrinth of interconnected corridors and ramps. The hallways were massively wide. Feeding off of them were narrower hallways that led to other parts, and the entire setup reminded one of a rabbit's warren den. This Friday night found them nearly void of people. Lost in thought, I took a wrong turn now I was also lost in the hospital. I was at a dead end in what started to feel like a rabbit warren and a sign told me I was in front of the morgue. I turned on a heel and ran, desperately seeking to return to some familiar sign. I stumbled into the main corridor and needed a few deep breaths before I could manage a very insincere laugh at my visceral reaction to being lost in a hallway and finding the morgue.

I finally got my bearings, and found the admissions department. Maybe this was not going to be so bad after all, I told myself. Surgery was necessary on this Friday night because cancer cells come in various types and can spread quickly. Some cells and tumors stay in the lymph nodes and other parts of the body for years and never grow; they are the pictures of self-contrast, the "benign" tumor. They never disperse and never intrude on the body's functions. Other cancer cells divide and grow immediately. Fox's strategy was to remove the apparent tumor with great haste. I walked the hallways alone before I called Debra.

I knew she could not come to the hospital right now. Sean was eight years old and Jeffrey was only three, and she had to be at home for them. First I called a friend at work to arrange for the boys to stay for the night, then phoned Debra so that I could offer a plan to make it easier for her to drop them off and be with me at the hospital. I collected myself, got my breath, and then dialed the number for my home.

"Hello." Her voice was bright and warm, relaxed. That was good.

"Deb? How are you doing'?" I was testing the waters on both ends of the line, putting special effort into hearing my own tone of voice.

"I'm fine, honey. What's up, Mark?" Unknown to either of us at the time, a border between us began.

I felt her words fall into a new but very discernible pattern. They hung between us, much like the first grains of sand are left ashore by waves at high tide, setting the patterns that some can see, and some cannot. Later, the words and ideas would grow and would build, as the ceaseless movement would leave more and more between us. All the while building a kind of perimeter fence around my loneliness in the disease. Debra began to see the wall growing between us before I did. But that would come later. From now, she simply spoke the words. "What is wrong? What is the mater?"

How to answer.

"I don't want you to worry, but we I'm at the hospital."

"Why Mark, what's the matter?" Another pregnant moment gave me time to both gauge her reactions and for me to gather some courage.

"I'm here at the hospital. I went to the doctor today for my physical and he says I need to go in for surgery on my testicle, tonight." The words came out with more ease than I expected, but my voice was beginning to crack at the edges.

"What did you say, Mark? What did *they* say? Honey what's wrong?"

"Well, he said it is probably cancer. They need to take out the testicle tonight and get a biopsy first thing tomorrow; he said every day counts in this kind of thing."

It was the first time I used the word. It stuck in my throat, then crept out slowly and meekly, like an unwanted guest. Can cer. Cans her. Her cancer? I said, heard, and actually felt the word. Then I added that I had already called some friends who would watch the boys that night.

"I'll be right there as soon as I can. What do you want me to do?"

There it was, the terribly hardest of questions: What can you do when someone you love says they have cancer? That question would haunt us from this day forward.

Her voice was cracking at the edges. She was trying to be brave, but I sensed she was barely under control. I decided to cut the tension.

"You can bring me some hard candy, my shaving kit, a book--that one on climbing, oh, and some clean underwear. You know how you always warn me to keep clean underwear or I'll be sorry for it. Well, you were right. About a dozen people today got to see my dirty underwear."

"The doctor saw your dirty underwear? I'm embarrassed.

"You're embarrassed? What about me? I'm the one who had to keep showing his testicles to different doctors all afternoon, one of which is a lady, trying to hide my underwear while doing it. Think about that."

We laughed while we cried. I told her I loved her, and hung up.

I thought that my strength of will and my physical responses to challenges were enough to carry me through any crisis. But my first emotions upon learning of the cancer were not about myself, but about my wife. Thoughts of me always occurred to me last. I wondered out loud and in explicit words about why I was like that, never seeking my own welfare and pleasure first. I thought I could handle it alone, but I wondered about her. I always held a little back from her. The delayed call represented many things that I had not learned to share with my wife yet. One of the healthy results that came from this night in 1987 was that I now began to openly share my innermost feelings with her. But on that night, I walked the halls alone until she arrived.

Medically, the decision to perform surgery was routine, very logical. It was straight line thinking: see a lump or a bump, diagnose, and cut it out. Deal with the personal conditions later.

But in personal and human terms, it was about as shocking and frightening as anything I could imagine. As much as this should have been all about me, about my testicle and my potential tumor, I felt strangely apart from, almost incidental to the process. I certainly did not get the idea that I was central to the events that began with great haste. It seemed a simple enough process, but I learned very soon that this was only the first step on a long road. The first steps, decidedly medical, were determined by the doctor. Very soon, however, the patient determines the course. I began this journey believing that my character was neutral to the outcome.

Fights against cancer are struggles against living enemies that feed on a body's systems. There were times when I knew that my cancer had gone crazy, that my body had revolted, and I thought that these out-of-control cells had developed human characteristics. They could sense, act, even think and plot against me. I thought the disease could read my mind, know the things I feared, and determine how to slowly and deliberately destroy me in the cruelest of ways: from the inside out. It found its way into the vulnerable areas.

But for now, I knew nothing of this ensuing war inside me. I was simply drinking the horrible tasting concoction the nurse fed to me that was supposed to empty my intestines. I had the terrible feeling it was about to go to work with a vengeance when my beautiful wife showed up at my bedside, looking at me dressed in a hospital gown sipping something through a soda straw.

"Hi. Want some? It's really good," I said in a comedy voice reserved only for her.

She didn't say anything. Just smiled and hugged me.

"Hi." she said, "Well what did they say?"

"They said I should find a better laundry," I joked.

She forced a small laugh while I added, "there really isn't much too it so far. They need to cut out the testicle to see what the growth is. Maybe it's cancer, maybe not. Don't worry too much. I still have another one."

Even less humorous. She just looked at me again.

"Deb, do you have a magic marker?

"A what?"

"I need to mark the side of the side so they don't take out the good one."

Finally she laughed.

The preparation called for cleansing the intestines and drawing blood for tests, and deciding the kind and amount of anesthesia. It did not take very long, and Doctor Fox was able to begin at about midnight. It was not a complex procedure. An incision about four inches long into the lower abdominal area, enabling the surgeon to remove the suspicious testicle. After he examined it, he knew it was cancerous by the color, texture, and size of mass. He would next focus his inquiry to determine the type of cancer cell.

Fox finished the surgery; he told Debra that it looked to him like it was cancer. The next few days became an eternity. My fate was in the hands of people and procedures completely foreign to me. Debra had only her own instincts and wits to insist on details about procedure, tests, possible effects. The shock of the announcement by the surgeon rocked her back on her heels. While I dreamed in the relative oblivion of the anesthesia, she endured those first horribly frightening moments of fear that trapped her on convoluted pathways and that colored every aspect of her world. Fox told her what he saw and felt some minutes before in the sterility of the operating room; a sterility quite apart from the dirty and messy world we were now in, but that only one of us yet knew. While I had the benefit of sleep, she had to drive home alone with her fears.

When I awoke, I felt as though I were part of a conveyor belt moving at blinding speed that suddenly stopped. A sense of urgency was in everything associated with my day. Now, there was a general stillness and everyone and everything simply waited. The piece of the removed tissue would be examined, evaluated, and circulated and evaluated by several urologist and oncologists. The waiting started on Monday and lasted ten days.

Even if the physical appearance of a tumor is quite unmistakable, doctors can assess its potential growth rate only with a biopsy. Independent judgments about the nature of the cells take time, and the waiting was tense. Bill Fox and the other doctors explained that my mental outlook was important, though they could not say why. This was the first of many instances when I knew I should defer my feelings to those who know a lot about cancer, but never experienced it.

When the biopsy returned seven days later, Doctor Fox met with Debra and me. "The tissue is cancerous," he began. "But there is good news. We know it is seminoma, a form of testicular cancer we see frequently. We know how to treat it."

We had taken a liking to each other. Bill Fox was becoming a friend as well as a trusted surgeon. I sensed that he wanted me not just to recover, but to get well. He gave his Friday night over to my surgery not because he had to, but because he knew it would make a difference. Debra and I talked and I saw him looking at her, I asked how he got his commission. He was in ROTC and he went to the summer camp training when I helped train the cadets in 1976. I now remembered him. He was the honor graduate of the camp. We joked a bit, then I told him Debra was in that camp as well and they vaguely remembered each other.

"As cancer goes, Mark, if you are going to get it, you got the right kind. The treatment is clear. Take prophylactic radiation therapy to stop it from spreading, called prophylactic. And the outlook is bright, about ninety per cent have full recovery."

The diagnosis was surprisingly comforting. There was now a next step, a tactical plan, a means by which this enemy could be fought. That was the way it would continue for years: meetings filled with thoughts and small sentences that together provoked enormous consequences. Contradiction and paradox were there. I took strange comfort in plans and procedures that involved poisoning or cutting me. Radiation poisons the healthy as well as the sick parts of the area. It relies on the premise that the healthy cells will regenerate, and the cancer cells will not.

Despite medical and technical advances, cancer can be reduced to a combination of three main treatments: surgery, radiation, and chemotherapy. In many cases though, the only experiences common from one patient to the next are three treatments. The ways in which people react to the processes vary as much as people do. Each step, whether a major meeting with doctors or a simple blood test with a nurse, seemed to put my course further out of my control. So I gave up trying to find control, and I instead followed orders.

I agreed to a test called a "lymphangiagram." It involved a surgical procedure designed to "read" the lymphatic system. It begins with large needles inserted between each toe, followed by the injection of a purple dye into the capillaries. The lymphatic system then filters the dye out of the blood making the entire lymphatic system visible by x-rays. The patient then waits for about two hours for the dye to move through the system, all to take x-ray pictures of the entire system.

The test was painful, not essential, and it held some measure of risk. But I elected to narrow the possibilities of where the cancer had spread. The clock measured two hours while the dye circulated thorough my system. If a standardized test such as a lymphangiagram exists, then why guess at the patient's status? I

may have been a humorous sight, and some might have
considered the lymphangiagram ridiculous, but I was not
compulsive. Without standardizing such a test, doctors and the
system unwittingly communicate that the patient will be OK
based on the previous population of patients, and the particular
study the treatment facility happens to follow. At a time of great
vulnerability, I was offered a very thorough picture of my
internal systems.

When I was sufficiently healed from the incisions on my
feet, and the lymphangiagram proved negative, Bill Fox turned
me over to a doctor in the radiology department, and we began
new planning sessions about the first steps for radiation therapy.
The physicians gave me the impression that my attitude would
be a central part of the treatment, but no one could explain this
vague generality about why it was so or elaborate on what I
should do. They did not know why or how. They just knew what.
They did not offer me any explanations. There were no
predictive models. There was very little discussion of "if we do
this, then that will happen," or anything like it. The radiologist
would not say how sick I would become, nor if any effects
would last. She did explain fully that the radiation would kill all
cells in the radiated area, a relatively large field from my
stomach to chest. While the healthy cells would regenerate in
about twenty-four hours the cancer cells would be killed. It was a
clear enough plan, just keep knocking down the enemy. But it
was never clear about how I would react.

I did not react well. Seminoma cells die when exposed to a
particular range of "rads," or radiation administered dose, the
measure of radioisotopes. But part of me died, too. My dose rate
was 115 rads for each daily treatment, for twenty-seven days, or
a total rate of 3,105 rads. *Mosby's Pocket Dictionary of
Medicine, Nursing, and Allied Health* defines radiation therapy
or *radiotherapy* as

...the treatment of neoplastic disease by using x-rays or gamma rays, usually from a cobalt source, to deter the proliferation of malignant cells by decreasing the rate of mitosis or impairing DNA synthesis.

Simply put, the patient is exposed to a "controllable" form of radiation poisoning.

I was neither emotionally nor mentally prepared for "therapy." When the doctors talked to me about the treatments, there was no mention of any mental and emotional side effects. We discussed only how the radiation affects the cells. I discovered that the non-physical aspects of the disease and the treatment would be left to me to resolve. Despite the lack of mental conditioning, I physically prepared in exact compliance with the standardized instructions. The first step was an interview and a tattoo session with the radiologist. She inked four dots permanently onto my abdomen, outlining a perfect rectangle. This defined a field that covered my intestines.

The radiation clinic held the contrast of upbeat and positive-minded people who dutifully tried to cheer up the patients as they prepared to bombard them with radiation poisoning. Despite the expectation that treatment processes are certain, techniques are imprecise. Radiation as "therapy" remains a relatively blunt instrument of medicine.

"Do you want to keep your remaining testicle safe from the therapy?" the radiologist asked me with no particular explanation or emotion.

The bizarre words caused me to laugh. "You're asking me?" I said in my best New York sarcasm. "I thought you were supposed to know that. We played twenty questions for a while. She asked if I still wanted more children, and I felt a little ill at ease. I knew there was another, less obvious reason for the question; that radiating the healthy testicle would render it not only sterile, but also vulnerable to new forms of cancer brought on by the treatments. But since there was no proof of such characteristics ascribed to radiation, we could not discuss it.

My instincts told me that I should protect the other testicle from radiation not because of sterility, but simply because my body was under enough stress already. What struck me later, however, was the weight of that decision. Although testicular cancer is the most common form of cancer in men, there is little open discussion about what men should consider when faced with it. My choice made, the radiologist explained that she could design a custom fit lead ball, complete with a slot to fit around my scrotum, so that the testicle would be protected from the radiation. It weighed about twelve pounds, and was cut exactly in half so that it could be fit around me. I would lie back on the table and await orders. Protected behind lead and glass shields, she would instruct me through different positions. "Turn on your left side.. Hold your breath...good." The machine buzzed, whirred, and clicked, then it was over. Thirty seconds. Back into the dressing room, take off the gown, and get dressed, then raced to the car to get home in time to fight the nausea. The radiologist, the two orderlies and I usually erupted in laughter at least once a morning while everyone coached me as to how to hold the lead ball over my testicle and wiggling the other parts of my body to fit the map now on my mid-section. Then the doctor would come in and carefully examine the graded field from my chest down to the groin. All of this happened in a surrealistic setting of a dark room with red and green rays and dots of light.

I joked with the orderlies while they prepared my "guardian ball," as they called it. It was a very strange looking object. I should have convinced them to let me keep it as a souvenir. It, or something like it, might very well be in some museum as a display of archaic medical practices in the ancient world.

My drives home were races against the clock of the inevitable nausea. The house would be empty; Debra was teaching pre-school. Jeffrey was with her, and Sean was in the third grade. I sat down and closed my eyes, trying to stop the spinning world. Spinning not as on a rope in climbing, but spinning like a top, like something thrown from afar and in a new place. My body was in the worst kind of war, the internal conflict that battles itself. The fires raged every day, always the same, an hour after return. The sickness would overwhelm in a way I thought not possible. My intestines, stricken once again assaulted, revolted after I got home, screaming and wailing in pain. They tightened and convulsed, and I could do nothing about it. There was no resistance left to the onslaught of the sickness. It washed over me first in the bowels and then in the gut, causing me to first undergo debilitating diarrhea, then vomit from deep within my intestines. I did not know that a person could vomit and undergo diarrhea at once.

When I began to vomit, it was violent and unrelenting. From the base of my spine to my throat, I controlled nothing. I gasped for air and my entire body was in a cold sweat and every muscle was engaged, generally in a contraction. It felt like every nerve ending was bared. With every session, I longed to run away, to retreat into my room, to flee. So afraid of that machine, so fearsome a thing it was to me. It was the source of so much sickness and pain. The little games I played in the first few sessions of treatment no longer amused. All I had was the sickness and the compelling need to flee the machines, the smells, the sights. I wanted fresh air, filled with rain, filled with the songs of birds and the scents of pine. I wanted air so different from the air of this room.

My patterns would continue as I awoke again and experienced unimaginable weakness, and again the building nausea, and once more no control at all, the source clearly deep within my intestines, within me, clearly not within my thinking or my subconscious, for I was completely ignorant at the time of the forces in chemistry that were raging out theories of equations and reactions within my cells. I was, in a phrase, at the mercy of the system. This was punishment for no crime.

By four o'clock each afternoon, the spinning in my head would slow enough to allow me some rest. I would sit and breathe slowly, then crawl into bed, dreading the next morning. For brief times, I would feel surprisingly strong, and when that occurred I felt compelled to spend time with my boys. On one particular occasion, I was strong enough to take Jeffrey to a lake, then to lunch at a nearby restaurant. The odors overwhelmed me, and I rushed home in blinding pain, my body revolting against the noises, odors, and tastes of what we call "normal" food in a busy restaurant. My entire sensory system seemed under assault. Even with nothing left to come up, the intestines revolted, enhancing the pain to new levels. My boys would grow accustomed to seeing me sick for some time, and quietly, diligently, with the same intestinal fortitude as the boxer of years before, I decided to fight this thing at its own level. I decided that whatever my kids would see, they would also see me fight back, maybe not today, but they would see it.

The waiting room for radiation therapy presents a great leveling effect. As hard as the physical parts of radiation sickness were, they paled in comparison to the emotional strains. In the waiting room of the radiology clinic, I discovered one of the hidden worlds of cancer patients. People waiting for radiation treatment are cautious, at first, about how to communicate with others. They come in all ages. Some look quite healthy. Some do not. Appearances disclose little. Most people just sit. They pretend to read, but actually they don't read much, because they physically cannot focus very well. Most people are very pleasant and very patient. Everyone seems to know that everyone else has got a serious problem. It may be very small, it may be life threatening, but in the waiting there is a great leveling effect. One morning, I noticed an older man. It occurred to me that we generally think of cancer patients as old, and this man fit the picture that most have. But next to him was a couple who was a little younger than Debra and me. They were with their ten-year-old child, a little girl who was in chemotherapy for some form of cancer that I no longer recall. The little girl asked me if I was sick. I told her I was, just a little, and asked her about herself and how she was. She quietly told me that she was sick and that she would probably not get better. But she came to the clinic to make the pain go away. And so the conversation went. Quiet small talk between adult and innocent child. Much like any other conversation between people who meet children and care to communicate with them; except that talks in hospital waiting rooms like this one room can easily shift to serious subjects like real life and real death.

I once worked with a Sergeant Major who had lost his young wife to cancer. He saw my reaction to chemotherapy two years later, and he told me this short story: "There is an enemy in there, somewhere. We think he's in the blood and the bone marrow. The doctors attacked his base camp, where he had a lot of strength, and they think they got most of them. We know the camp is gone. Destroyed the camp. But these guys may have gotten away and we don't know just where they are. So we act like a wolverine. We soil it so badly in all the places he might hide that even if there are some of them left, they have no where to live. We measure how well this tactic works by what the friendly forces (the white blood cells) in the area tell us. We move all friendly forces out for a while, even though we need them. We'll get them back later, when it's all clear. "

He invented private metaphors for the things he feared. The man's story dealt with the insanity of cells gone crazy in our own

ways. His tone and humor compelled me to look in the mirror.
He knew the complexities of what actual cells were really at
work in his wife's lymphatic system. He just could not talk about
them in precise medical terms. He used words common to his
own remarkable experiences. He also expressed a great respect
for the disease itself and a great love for the brave lady who
fought the hard fight but then simply had to rest. He never
expressed winners or losers in his story of the fight. He never
cursed his enemy the disease. In fact, he accepted it. Left with
three children, two still at home, and a lifetime of habits that had
not prepared him for his new role as single parent. He adjusted.
One of the ways he assigned meaning to his young wife's death
was with this little story. It was medically simple, but accurate.
Some of the enemy just got away and came back and ambushed
her.

One day when Jeffrey was home with me I got very weak
and sick and I had to lie down. As I dozed, I heard the door slam
and I sensed that he had left the house. I leapt from the sofa and
the pain in my head threw me to the floor. I fought through it and
managed to grab a coat to cover my bare and frail body as I
plunged into the Northwest cloud that filled the day outside my
door. I could not see him and could not muster the strength of
voice to call him. So I somehow ran down the street, hoping and
praying I would not collapse. I caught him just as he was about
to enter a main road. He just looked at me and smiled as if we
were playing a we playing a kind of game. I carried him back to
the house and doubled up in pain as I deposited him inside the
doorway. I stood out in the rain and gasped for air. I vomited. I
wondered out loud how much more of this I could tolerate, how
much more before I would be myself again. But I missed the
essential point. It was what I saw as I gazed in the mirror, and
the terribly debilitating sight of weakness, which was, for a time

at least, my new self. I had been transformed for a purpose I could not yet see.

Sean was eight years old. He was just able to understand enough of all this to be afraid. I do not know when children become afraid of the real world. There was more than enough fear and uncertainty in the world to worry about children's fantasies. I don't know when children understand words like cancer and death, but Sean, at eight, knew them well. While I was in radiation treatment, he avoided any talk of what might be wrong with me. Children at school first questioned, then teased him, about what had happened to me, about what kind of cancer I had. At some point, he probably told one of his classmates that my tumor was of the testicle and then the teasing began. It was a hard way to discover the special cruelty that is a part of childhood.

Somewhere in this time, he began taking his feelings and setting them aside. He stopped talking about how he felt. He stopped asking how I felt. As the weeks passed, time seemed to support what I told my son. I looked a little better with each passing day. The effects of radiation subsided, and I started to talk about the cancer as if it were over and would never be back. In other words, I did not discuss it at all.

Debra could not convince me to face the cancer. I chose to consider it "over." She cajoled, described, read, and discussed, but I would not listen. I simply did not want to think about it. I began to go out alone, enjoyed days by myself. I had no plans, no ideas on what must be or what should be. I made no judgments. In the weeks after the radiation treatment, my ideas about time were undergoing amazing transformation. It simply did not matter whether it was lunch or dinnertime, this or that time. What mattered was what I need needed or wanted to do. For the first time in my life, I was free of the clock and the calendar. But was I "free of disease?"

Reality returned with the first set of Computer Tomography scans. The process produces circular x-ray pictures of the body. Most patients take CT scans every three to six months. I prepared for the event by drinking the two quarts of licorice flavored contrast liquid to insure that the x-rays and the contrast could be readable. I found it ironic that licorice is the only flavor I really don't like. I gagged it down. Then, with arms extended back over my head, the intravenous tube enters the vein. There was a strong, medicinal, hot sensation, first in my arms, then moving slowly to my chest, and eventually to my abdomen. My ears and nose and face were on fire. The machine sounded like a muted dishwasher, a rotating, rhythmic noise that penetrated my entire body. The pattern of it has become etched in my memory, and any similar noise returns my mind to the scan machine.

The purpose of the CT's is to detect any growths and densities that might develop in the tests. It is as if one is looking down through the top of my head, and every five centimeters, you see a complete x-ray view of all organs from that perspective so the overall effect is to thinly slice through the body to see if anything abnormal is hidden anywhere.

With each small part of treatment, I was becoming more captured by the process, and I was becoming strangely comfortable with it. I did not yet see the need for introspection and self-direction. I avoided any questioning about just why I believed I got the cancer. After all of the pain of the radiation and now the further probes of the CT process, did I continue to believe a little too much in the words of the diagnoses? Words and phrases like "benign," "mild form of cancer," "very treatable," and "free of disease" were beginning to conflict with my short, but nonetheless intense experiences with cancer. I wanted to consider the cancer a temporary condition, something that I could handle with the right physical steps. I wanted it to pass.

I am not sure what led me to the misguided idea that this was all about some test of myself that only I could pass or fail, but I know now that I considered my family only incidental to the cancer.

In my office hangs a poster-sized photograph that I took during one of my climbs in Mount Rainier National Park. Mount Rainier is the centerpiece of the dramatically beautiful Cascade Mountain range in Washington State. Only an experienced eye would find something peculiar about the scene. If the day held a summit assault, then why is the 4,412 foot domed peak in the picture? And what is that cloud? The radiation treatments ended in March, and in May I decided to climb again. The three-day adventure occurred about six weeks after my radiation sessions ended. Elliott Gruner, one of my closest friends, an exceptional athlete and mountaineer, agreed to go with me. It was June and the funnel cloud began about one thousand feet above Rainier's dome and rises at least five thousand feet higher. The sky is deeply blue and very calm all around the massive mountain. We could not see this cloud coming. It came from the far side of the crest, from the east. The Nisqually Indians called Rainier "TA-HO-MA," or snow covered mystery. Northwest volcanic mountains have a distinctive "lenticular" shaped cloud that caps the domed peaks. While its shape does not indicate any movement to the untrained eye, it can dissipate on the leeward side while forming on the windward, and the effect can be sixty mile per hour winds under perfectly clear blue sky. On this day, the cloud was all that went wrong, but it was quite enough. The winds approached one hundred miles per hour.

I did something that day I had never done before. I let go of the goal and surrendered to the conditions, We left the ascent to the domed peak and found a different, lower climb on Unicorn Peak in the Tatoosh Range. I have since focused not on the peak of Rainier in that beautiful photograph, but instead on the cloud.

One part of my eventual successful fight against cancer was to accept the many failures that accompany the disease. This is a story not only of success, but of failure. I needed the failures so that I might change. I had to begin to look in the mirror differently and see that my battles were inside. I had to find a different way to think about it. Whether I changed my outlook or not, my body had been transformed, and it would never be the same as it was before.

When the great comedian Sid Caesar was inducted into the Comedy Hall of Fame, he had a timeless message...

"Everybody has a now. All of us have them, everyone. It doesn't matter how much or little you have. We all have a now. But none of us can keep a now. Nows turn very quickly into wuzzes. There is nothing you can do about it. A now becomes a wuzz. Period...

These wuzzes, you have to watch them... If you don't, they can become very heavy. They can hang around your neck and weigh you down. When that happens, they can turn into very bad wuzzes, ones that I call shoulda, coulda, woulda's. You don't want 'shoulda, coulda, woulda's.' They ruin many good times. You have to get rid of those.

...You also have to watch the wuzzes that they don't lead to gotta's and gonnas. 'Gotta's and Gonnas' cannot really be done, and trying to do them can make you very unhappy....

The thing to do is to take the wuzzes, keep the happy ones, and let the others go...Take the nows and make them count. Take the shoulda, coulda, wouldas, take the gonnas and gottas and let them go."

Although I did not think on my disease again for some time, I also did not consider such wise advice about the "shoulda, coulda, woulda's." I simply put it away.

My old life began in 1952 in the only part of New York City on the mainland of the United States, The Bronx. When I was born, my mother told me once, giving me a rare glimpse of her husband and only partner for thirty five years, my father held me up and told her I was going to go to West Point. I never thought much on that scene until many years later when as the father of two boys I thought about how dramatic, how rock solid an approach to life, how at once admirable and frightening that scene must have been for my mother. Both came from the city, grew up there, and their lives were very much a part of that unique and wonderful world called New York. My fathers' first and possibly most significant statement about me, his first son, was something a mother would not forget.

For my parents, much like millions of their time, life was good in the years following the war. In the early 1950s in New York as in most of the country, more work led to more earnings, which led to nest eggs and the American dream. For my father, though, the times were even more fundamental, almost philosophical. He had survived not only a war, but the war. He was not just there, not just incidental to the event, but a real part of it. He didn't wax philosophical. They put their family together, worked hard, told me and my brother and sister to study, and we learned by example.

World War II imprinted an indelible confidence on him. He was drafted into the horse cavalry and joined the famous 10th Mountain Division in Italy where he was a member of the mounted infantry reconnaissance squadron. He was among the last soldiers in the United States Army who went into battle on horseback. He would joke that when people would discover that he rode horses in the war, they complimented him for his young healthy looks. They thought he was a veteran of the first, not the Second World War. He fought as both a mounted infantryman on horseback and as a ski trooper. He told stories about how to keep horses quiet during ambushes and how to keep new lieutenants from using parade ground tactics and screaming "Charge!" with drawn sabers. He loved to entertain. Even as a catcher in softball, anyone who ever watched him play remembered not the power with which he hit the ball. Instead, they remember that incredible, loud, funny character behind home plate. No one was immune from his verbal abuse. He could actually make a story about each hitter and laugh at the top of his lungs. The catcher never ceased. My friends would ask if he was always like that. I never answered.

The roar of his power built the quiet parts of me.

To me, he was larger than life itself. He had the utmost, undying respect for the officer corps that led him into battle. He never went to college; his education came in other forms; and when he was drafted, he went with enthusiasm, taking charge in ways that could commend him for commissions, but he wanted none of it. He had his standards, and he knew that the officers required education that he did not have nor seek. So he was the best sergeant he could be. He was a man at once in touch with these times and with other times. His father died when he was seventeen years old and he spent his life at work, both before and after the war. He had only one thing to tell me about my future. Having told my mother where I would go to school at my birth, he told me a hundred times, "The best school in the world is fifty miles from here, West Point. If you really work, you'll go there."

My mother, like my father, grew up in the Bronx. Her parents owned a butcher shop, and although she told powerful stories of the Depression, she would openly allow that here childhood was very good for at least these reasons: parents who loved their children, a feeling of community despite the lack of money, and the simple fact that her father brought home food from his store.

When I was fifteen years old, and I wanted to train for a trip to Philmont Scout Ranch in New Mexico for an expedition of hiking and climbing for two weeks, she reluctantly agreed, even thought she felt I was too young. And two years later, when at the age of seventeen I was accepted for admission to West Point, she again agreed, this time with reluctance that only a mother can understand. In later years, she would tell me later that all through the application process she never believed that West Point would accept me, and even if they did that I would decline the appointment. I was only seventeen, she reasoned, and I would not really want to commit to the military for that many years.

My household was a great mix of ideas and viewpoints. A collection of argument, humor, healthy and some not so healthy tension. When Dad's salary improved, we moved when I was ten years old to Bronx Park East in the northern section of the borough. It seemed to be a world apart form the dense apartment buildings that we left on Boston Road and 174th Street, just a few miles away. It was the only time I moved.

As a child, I felt I had the benefit of two lives. One was in the city; the other was the summer in the country. I thought everyone got to do that. We would take summers in the Catskill Mountains, near Monticello, New York. The bungalow colonies attracted the same crowds each summer. My favorite place was called Anawana Beach Colony, on the beautiful lake by the same name, near a major hotel and sports camp. I would awake each morning at six, walk the mile or so to the golf course, and caddie.

One of my oldest friendships began at Evander Childs High School with Marc Guthartz. Evander was a typical New York City school of the day. Just beneath the surface of the rowdiness and noise was a love of teaching and therefore an opportunity for learning. Marc and I learned a lot. It was hard to say good bye to Marc. He planned a surprise going away party for me. Until that night, I don't think West Point was a reality for me. I went there with youthful idealism, thinking and believing it was about patriotism. I could always hang on to Marc's friendship. In the tumultuous summer of 1969, at the age of seventeen, while some of my high school friends left their homes for Woodstock, I departed for West Point. Fifty miles and a world away from The Bronx. I was fascinated with what cadets from other parts of the country thought and did. It was an amazing collection to me, a cacophony of fast friends who were pitted against powerful upperclassmen.

I was the youngest man in my class. The first few weeks were hard on me, and the weight loss from the hazing in "Beast Barracks," cadet orientation and basic training, weakened my will. I wanted no help from outside, but when my mother came to visit me, she was so worried that she summoned my father from his reserve duty at Fort Drum, in distant upstate New York. When he walked into the cadet central guardroom in uniform, complete with combat ribbons and a presence the cadet guards probably sensed, they summoned me to see my father.

We walked to Trophy Point, and while overlooking the Hudson, surrounded by statues and monuments, symbols not only of graduates but of the professional officer corps, citizen soldier Bob Gerner tried to tell his son about how to engage this part of life under these kind of circumstances at the age of seventeen. I knew only that I wanted to succeed here, a week or a year at a time. He told me that if it became too much for me, then I should come home. "Don't stay here to prove something for your father. I'm more proud of you for having gotten here than you can know. I just don't want you hurt. If you are not ready for this, if this is not for you, give it up."

I decided then that I would not quit. The irony for me was that hearing I could come home made me more resolute than ever to succeed at this craziness called plebe year and graduate from whatever this school was. It was one of my earliest lessons, one forgotten and relearned many times over: we all carry baggage, and it changes very little over time, but the little bits that do change can matter a great deal.

They called it "character building" then. It is known by different labels now, but no matter what it is called, it continues to be the philosophy that successes of value are gained through some level of sacrifice. It is the most instructive windows into the growth at all levels that I have ever seen. I was quite fortunate to have gone there. In the summer of 1969, I was in trouble. It made for high stress, but also it made for high comedy. It tested us in ways that were quite deep and quite important. It was an American Sparta. Strength and courage were paramount, and no one ever expected that we would graduate.

We were told a lot, believed some of it, and though there was a lot to complain about, there was little complaining. It made for life long friends, of which I was fortunate to make many, but none occupied the same place as one Robert Miller. Born in France and educated in Europe, he was fascinated whit the United Sates, especially in New York City. He saw the city and loved it. He spent one of his summer leaves, only thirty days, driving a cab in Manhattan. Bob and I spent New Year's eve in Times Square in to usher in 1973. It was five below zero, and we were looking for the two sisters who lived in an apartment on the east eighties that we had dated together some months before. But we couldn't find the street, much less the apartment, and we ushered in the year with each other. Years late, when there was little left of me, Bob helped me find my way again. My interests varied as I grew up there, even finding a

singing and dancing part as a puppet maker in the "Hundredth
Night Show," a musical comedy show done by the seniors about
one hundred days before graduation.

While others struggled through only a required class and
spent the time on calculus to maintain some competitive form as
a plebe, I willingly joined the company gladiators on the boxing
team. Calculus mattered, but it carried not nearly the weight that
"fighting for the company" did. I was one of the gladiators on
the Corps-famous "Hawg One," or company H-1 boxing team.
The price of visible courage and proof of manhood can be high
at the age of seventeen. It was high for me, but it held its
rewards. The upper clansmen began to offer me some modicum
of respect. I had desperate for some privacy, and with each fight
and each letting of blood for "the company," I seemed to gain a
few more minutes each day. I liked the idea that I had finally
found something that made me feel strong and skilled at this
crazy place.

There was a day in my years there that stands apart. An
afternoon in Manhattan found my father and me in a rare
situation: alone together. It was May of my junior year and I was
in the city to march in the Armed Forces Day Parade on Fifth
Avenue. After, he took me to a late lunch, and for once there was
no rush to our apartment in the north Bronx. We had planned
that I would not stay overnight. I had to get back and study for
finals. I planned to walk across town to the usual pick up point
for the bus rides back up the Hudson, but that was several hours
and a lifetime of stories away from our lunch. He loved his
stories.

The light in the street was golden. It easily warmed city air
recently chilled by an early spring rain. The aromas of the
world's food encircled and swirled around us. He used to like to
tell me that our hometown belonged to the world. But it was
more than that to me, it was his city. The rare mix of scents of

trees, blossoming flowers, and freshly washed concrete tantalized with Italian sauces and German beer and bread. The day and the company were both distinctly New York, and it was the first time since I had gone away to the Academy that my father and I visited alone.

Somewhere in our visit, I gained the comfortable feeling that he looked upon me as an adult. In the years when the Vietnam War was central to life in the Army, living within the stone gray walls of the fortress West Point removed us from many of the debates of the day. There was then, as there remains now, some merit in keeping the future officer corps apart from issues such as the moral basis of a war, the connections between local political and foreign policy. And many other painful and controversial subjects of the day. Our professional education was not about controversy. It was about duty, honor, country, period.

Whatever the rationale, we felt quite apart form the Vietnam War. It was clear that the war had become very central to the Army, yet it was also clear that for me and the future officers of my time, the Vietnam War was moving to an almost incidental importance, almost as if it did not happen. I found the contrast fascinating. I thought that if anyone would be included in the what and why of the Vietnam War, it would be West Point cadets. Yet there was virtually nothing in our experience there to connect any of us to the looming war in Vietnam.

I wanted to know about soldiers in combat, and all I could gather from the time was how vastly different Vietnam was from World War II. Now, with our better trained ears and our advantages of hindsight and personal maturity, we can see that the human element of behavior in war is relatively constant. The changes in each generation's wars are not in how soldiers behave or the life and death struggles they face, but rather the changes are in what we do with the wars, how we receive the experiences back into our fabric of society. The emotions and humanity that accompany war: cruelty, heroics, humanity, and yes love, what happens there is as it has always been. What we do with it collectively and politically changes dramatically, even as much as what we do technologically. My father understood these notions and he answered my need to know about battle with a story about his horse.

If you listened carefully when my father spoke, you heard love stories.

His reconnaissance patrol was sighted by an enemy observation post high above the Po Valley in the Italian Alps, and the artillery rained in. Sergeant Gerner, normally very skilled and adept in both horsemanship and soldiering, was adrift on the field. He began his tale.

> *...It started with the artillery. You just couldn't get away from it, no matter how you might expect it, no matter what you did. And with horses...well, it was just a little crazy.*

I sat in silence, mystified. I wanted to pinch myself and wondered if he was talking to me or if he had spotted some reporter who was doing a feature for the Sunday Times.

> *...the artillery did not stop. I was hoping it would be just a few rounds, but it was clear they had us spotted and stuck. I wanted to help the lieutenant and the platoon, but first I had to get my horse under control, so I dismounted and covered her head. I cradled her and soothed her by whispering in her ear, trying to control the panic, but it was no good. She wasn't suffering from panic of the noise, but from wounds. There was crying and shouting and horses and mules were making such a racket and nearly trampling us, it was almost funny. I looked for the place to go, you can normally spot some place where the shells are not falling,*

but with the horse, well you had to be careful before getting them up. I picked out a spot and got her up, then I saw the broken hoof and all the blood. I left her and made my way to the aid station. I had to find the Doc..

But he could not do anything, and I had to destroy her.

A horse, an innocent animal, should not die like that, it shouldn't die because men are trying to kill other men. In battle, just remember that your men will look to you for the humanity. Not many people will tell you that, but it's true. Men will see and do things they will never do outside of battle and they will expect their officers to remind them that they are human and that humanity matters. Men will make mistakes and you will make mistakes, but hang on to your humanity.

I remember looking at him and thinking that it was an answer to a question I did not ask, but then his expression, his unforgettable smile told me to just take it in and trust him. The story now over, so was the day. As we parted, he for his drive up to the Bronx and me to the west side to find the buses back to West Point, his voice suddenly became light hearted,

"A man gets a different view of the world form the top of a horse... A better view."

Anxious to get started in the Army, I made my way to Fort Lewis for my first assignment. I was like a sponge in what I learned. I never attached any great higher meaning to the troops and to the training, I just liked it. The Pacific Northwest, its climate, the mountains, the skiing, the cities of Seattle and Tacoma, the people. All of it made me quite comfortable. They struck me as friendly and accepting, generally operating with a

quiet and understanding attitude of 'live and let live.' I was
twenty-one years old, and the world awaited me.

Three years later, in the summer of 1976, I met Debra on a
rifle range on Fort Lewis. She was an ROTC cadet at summer
training. A romantic beginning, we both surrendered, all reason
would have told us that it would never last, just too different. She
had decided that the Army was not for her. She hated to take
orders, and the Army had little to do with her goal: teaching
children. She was also stunningly beautiful with large brown
eyes, long legs, and wonderfully dark brown hair. We stayed
engaged for a year while awaiting her graduation from Utah
State University. We were married at her home in Logan, Utah,
in May of 1977. That is when our families met. Having attended
our wedding, many of my friends are probably not surprised that
I survived two tests of cancer, after I survived the Bronx, New
York meeting Logan, Utah.

The last time I saw him alive was at our wedding. He had so
much fun visiting Logan Utah and meeting Deb's father. Debra
and I were married in May of 1977. Sean was born in July 1978,
and the heart attack that changed all our lives came August of
1978. Just when I was a beginning to see his wisdom while I was
a rifle company commander and I would think about how much
he loved me, death took him, and when it did, it took a part of
me also. It shook my foundation until it rattled; it may even have
cracked. It took my humor. At the age of twenty-six, I learned
we are mortal.

Death and Bob Gerner simply did not go together.

Debra's fist view of New York's skyline was from the
Newark Airport at two in the morning with four week old Sean
in her arms. We drove the rental car up through New Jersey,
crossed over to the New York State Thruway to Route 17 toward
Monticello, the place of so many fond summers for me as a boy.
The familiar country roads, embedded in my memory form so

many Friday nights, awaiting my father to make the very same drive up to the cottage after his long week at work in the city's summer heat. The same landmarks were there, and the car nearly navigated itself in my hands. A short way out of the town was the Lake Anawana, the site of where we spent so many summers and now the site where my father fell out of the car the night before, just before he died in the hospital.

Early the next morning, we all drove back to the city and began the arrangements.

It was a blur, and none of it mattered very much. The days left me exhausted, emotionally drained. Those terribly simple yet amazingly difficult tasks of death; the plot the service, the money, the casket, the phone arrangements, the flowers, and the eating. All of it was upon us, either my brother, myself, or some relative. The arguments raged as my mother could not decide what detail she needed to attend to before or after which, and I just ran on adrenaline and wondered where he was. We cleanse ourselves of the dead, banishing them to places away from our existential world, and we try to set them apart not so much to remember them but to free ourselves. "Funerals are for the living," my friend Marc told me, and he was right. But it would take me years and my own cancer to accept that.

That was 1978. The years between his death and my first case of cancer were filled with the excitement and the adventure that career in the infantry can offer, and filled with the love of my wife and two great sons. But all of my times are overshadowed by these two moments: his death and my first case of cancer. Nine years after my father's death, I was still trying to get in touch with my own sense of mortality and humanity. I scaled a peak, yes, but I did not yet understand the connections of the climb. My first experience with testicular cancer was not an encounter, but only a brush, a passing glance, with a serious disease. If I looked upon it all, I did so wrongly. I thought I was in a direct, physical fight, something that was now over. And a t that time, my fighting was predictable, straight ahead.

My trip to Mount Rainier on that memorable day between cancers offered me clues, brief images of my strength, set in between seemingly endless episodes of sickness. The margins of my illness were barely visible to me. None of the scene would focus, not until much later. Meanwhile, my trails traveled only physical and topographic crests while I grew thirsty for other kinds of summits.

3 MOMENTS

*Cancer: ...a malignant invasive cellular tumor that has
the capability of spreading throughout the body or body
parts. Microbiology by Tortoa, Funke and Case.*

*Abnormal cell division: ...when cells in some area of the
body divide without control, the excess of the tissue that
develops is called a tumor, growth, or neoplasm. The study
of tumors is called oncology. (onco = swelling or mass;
logos = study of). A cancerous growth is called a malignant
tumor or malignancy. A noncancerous growth is called a
benign tumor.* Principles of Anatomy and Physiology by
Tortora and Grabowski.

Men who get testicular cancer generally recover with only
minor limitations. One measure of recovery is the statistics, and
like all such numbers, they drive us toward predisposed notions
and confirm what we mostly know or want to conclude anyway.
Out of both desperation and hope, I sought some education in the
data, but I found little. With testicular cancer of the seminoma
variety, the data suggest that only about ten per cent of all cases
return, and if the cancer comes back, it is in a treatable form.
Cancer moves through the lymph system into nodes of the lower

abdomen and possibly as far away as the chest. My case fit the pattern seminoma so well that it seemed a foregone conclusion I would never again suffer any real consequences. The less I considered cancer, I reasoned, the faster it would be over.

I thought the entire episode was misplaced, an anachronism that would somehow correct itself in time. I had taken a short trip into the world of the sick, but I was back now and I had no need to worry. I saw little need to consider the disease; it was like a drive from New England to Georgia on Interstate 95. Look out the window while passing through the South Bronx and then claim you have been there. But there was no need to stay long. This place of cancer had little to do with me, not in any personal ways. It was nothing more than a brief encounter.

Now late in May, two months after the completion of radiation, I was assigned as the executive officer of an infantry battalion. Our unit would soon go on a peacekeeping mission as part of the Multinational Force and Observers, the military organization that enforces the peace between Israel and Egypt in the Sinai desert. But before I could take the new assignment I had to appear before a medical board that would evaluate my potential for future service. I collected the required letters that stated I was a good officer and should remain in the Army, but I had no enthusiasm for all the bureaucratic and administrative connections to this. I just wanted to go to work.

At the age of thirty-five, I was still naive about the forces that can shatter a life. I still believed that with work and will I could control my own destiny. But when I appeared before the board, I got a different view. In the waiting room was a quiet man of about my age, a sergeant. He moved around with a slight limp, and he nervously clung to some papers. His eyes begged me to start the conversation.

"How are you doing?" I asked quietly.

"O.K., I guess. They still don't know what's wrong with me. I got hurt about a year ago. The pain in my neck and back never stop." My "What happened?" triggered a story.

He began with the earnest slow talk that seems to be at least the invention, if not the private property, of people who work hard for a living. "I was under a truck and I turned and something just cracked in my back. Never been the same since. I can't carry on like this. I just can't be in the Army and not work. I'm too proud for that. The medical people have been real good and tried to help, but they say my condition will never change. Something I can't pronounce. I really like the Army. Been a soldier for fifteen years. It's all I know, and I'm trying hard to stay, but I just don't know."

He talked about his wife and children with great love. His easy drawl put him somewhere from the South. He was a good man. He was suddenly done and he asked me a simple question, "Sir, are you going to be OK?"

His words riveted me. They were shocks of super cooled arctic air. I felt like I did in an Alaskan tundra in December when I passed the barrier of a warm arctic tent into the still air of forty below at four in the morning. All moisture freezes, the body does not breathe, and everything shuts down for a few seconds. I had not yet made the connections between cancer and death. I did not yet realize why and how cancer could make one wish for death. When death comes, it can be the great relief because the cancer does not kill until some vital organ, such as the liver or spleen is so interwoven with the disease that it simply fails. It is either that or the other, more weakening condition where the body simply starves. My kind of cancer was not connected to death, it was just one of those "little" cancers.

But the tone and the tense of his question bothered me. How I will be. It may have been the first time that I thought about the future.

About one per cent of men get testicular cancer. It usually occurs between the ages of nineteen and thirty-five, and is normally very treatable, meaning that doctors can predict the behavior of the types of cells that form its tumors. Medical statistics, wrapped up in the social fabric so filled with other trends and numbers that provide a sense of comfort than they do a warning about a dangerous state. Just as the statistical chances of traffic accidents do not lock people in their homes, the statistical chances of cancer do not limit people's actions until a tumor invades. Abundant rationalizations keep the tumors away from our doors and away from our bodies.

The icy blast of his question left me as I reasoned that I must be well.

"Yes. I'm sure I will be. I did have cancer, but now I'm fine," I said unconvincingly.

"You beat it so far. That's great. I hope you make it."

Someone called his name, and as we parted his expression changed just at the edge, just enough to show fear rather than confidence. Fifteen minutes later he walked out, shaken. He quietly said that the board would recommend dismissal with disability. His hands looked strong and gritty, worn like leather. They clutched at his small collection of letters, held them as if they strung together in a lifeline. It looked as though this was the first time he thought about leaving the Army. Each letter was signed by previous commanders or other officers in whom he invested great faith. Though I never met him before and would never see him again, he made a permanent impression, the image of the faithful soldier dismissed, not rejected or shunned, but dismissed nonetheless. The process is fair enough. A higher board would certainly award some level of disability, but that was not the issue for this man on this day. Instead, he was reviewing his value as a person. As he wished me luck and said good bye, his tearful eyes stayed on the letters.

I walked into the room, brought myself to the position of attention and saluted smartly, formally reporting to the president of the board. I took my seat in the chair positioned in the middle of the room, and I realized I had never before been officially "on the spot" in quite this way. Every face but one was familiar. Physical Evaluation Boards are comprised of field grade officers, majors and lieutenant colonels. Members of the board must be senior to the soldier under consideration, and since I was a major, the board members were battalion commanders and they were, coincidentally, the commanders from the brigade in which I served. The one new face was that of the medical officer.

There were a few easy questions. "How do you feel?" "Are you back at physical training yet?" "Do you feel you can work a full day?" Everyone but the doctor seemed to be impressed with my appearance. The familiar faces and voices paid me some compliments. "I saw you running yesterday. You looked strong." Things like that. To the uninitiated, it appears that someone who looks fit is also healthy. Looks count for a lot.

The fact that I was now recovered to full physical strength, two months after the removal of one testicle and radiation treatment. The effects of radiation poisoning: vomiting, hair loss, scarring, and weight loss appear to last for only days after treatment ends. The long-term effects are still debated. Nonetheless, it provided something of a common language, this language of physical training between soldiers, so that we could open the board and have something to talk about. The discussion was professional, to the point, but also quite comfortable and informal. Only the doctor reserved on the point of my prospective health.

No one asked about my emotional state, about my family, about anything except my physical health and my duty performance. There was no mention of counseling or support groups, and especially no questions about my state of mind.

Under the provisions of the governing regulation, that would
have been fairly inappropriate in this process. Besides, they all
knew I was already back at work. This was, after all a "Physical
Evaluation Board." The doctor asked me if I understood the
importance of the tests that would follow. He mentioned that it
was possible, even somewhat likely, for these tumors to return.
Looks of disdain, particularly from me, answered his unwelcome
points of fact. The "profile," the medical condition signed by the
surgeons read "free of disease." What more did anyone need to
know? Was he, as a medical professional, suggesting that this
was not correct? Was this to suggest that I may not be healthy?
No, not at all, he explained. The medical record was very clear,
the outlook excellent. The doctor saw fit to remind me that this
was cancer, not some mole or infection, and that I needed to
understand it and to be careful. But there was no room on this
panel for any debate; these people knew that the right thing for
me was to return me to full duty so that I could deploy with my
unit to the Sinai, so that I could put this behind me and get on
with the ever important career. Ironically, the biggest champion
of this idea back then was me.

The board recommended that I remain on active duty. It also
noted that I should stay in the Infantry, and returned to full duty.
I had to keep the "P3" label for assignment limitations, until two
years passed. The profile's code means that the limitation is
"permanent" and it is in the "3" area of the body. The human
body is divided into logical areas by code. "P" means "physical
systems" and "3" means "significant limitations," which signals
the medical treatment facilities that the patient requires special
attention, possibly reclassification for duty. The purpose of this
was so that the Army could not assign me to an area where
cancer treatment was not available.

An irony began on this day that remains with me still. The
doctors had labeled "free" (Free of disease). The board validated

that code word with their conclusion and recommendations. But I was also fooled and imprisoned by my newly noted "freedom." I allowed the disease to get away that day, before I got to take it out and examine it for how it worked in me. So I got to cheat for a while. Without doing the hard work to examine and reject the cancer, I was allowed to simply set it aside. Despite the fact I had not yet faced it, I could now really call it "over," and I did.

Cancer's weapons in this battle were stealth and camouflage. It fooled the members of the board, and it especially fooled me. It deceived me into the belief that none of my behaviors were unhealthy and none of my thinking was wrong. Everything about me, my psychological makeup, my behavior, my character, my sense of spirituality, had no connection at all to cancer or to the disabilities of disease; and especially no connections to death. I beat this thing by just being myself. I think one of the incredibly puzzling and interesting things in disease is not that we fail to learn the lesson of it. I learn, forget, then learn again.

The doctors were cautious about how to advise me about my upcoming six month trip to the Sinai. They would have preferred I not go, but they also understood and supported me in my desire to do my job and continue my career. My follow-up treatment called for standardized tests every three months three blood tests: beta "HCG" and alpha pheta protein, two tumor markers, and testosterone levels. I also needed computer tomography scans, chest x-rays, and a physical examination. These tests in themselves do not tell a doctor that a patient has a returned case of cancer, behind the obvious tumor. Instead, there are sets of tests that when taken together serve as a series of gates, each filtering out some possibilities and offer up others. One end of the spectrum tells you complete health, one end leads you to near certainty you are looking at the behavior of a cancerous tumor. The doctors determined that I could get the same level of testing in Israel, so they cleared me to go on the mission. In my mind, this was all very routine.

Infantry battalions are naturally close knit, almost like extended families of the Army. The Third battalion, 47th Infantry was especially so. The months of preparation for the mission lasted over nine months. We had a large staff, and it would have been "good therapy" for any infantry officer. For me, it was perfect.

Debra and I knew how to express our "good-byes," but this time would be different. This took so much time to anticipate. In March, a few weeks before I left, we took a trip to Washington's stormy and remote coast on the Olympic Peninsula. We went to La Push, the very northwest tip of the state. Driving out to this tiny beach town in late March 1988 was like driving into a different time. The land remains as it always has been: raw and powerfully beautiful. The beaches are wide, long, and filled with debris of huge trees and the occasional crashed boat. The sand seems to entice incredibly powerful storms in to land. Clouds and the wind mix hard against the rocks. I nonetheless insisted that we go out and build the campfire we planned. We tried to seek shelter in between rocks and driftwood, huge pieces; they looked as if giants had tossed them like so many toothpicks. After a short time everyone was scampering back to the cabin. I wanted to breathe in the wind and the sea.

I looked up and saw my wife. I didn't expect her to stay out with me and especially didn't expect her to join me once she had gained the warmth of the cabin.

"What are you doing out here?" she asked.

"Looking for a date. How about you?"

"Well, I thought I saw some guy who looked kind of cute. But I must have been mistaken. Mark, Is something wrong?"

I shrugged. "I don't know, not really. I'm just a little mixed up. I hope I'm over all this with the cancer. But I don't know.

Maybe this trip is just what I need. But I really will miss you. And the boys. Are you sure you'll be OK?"

It was nearly a year since cancer and Debra and I still had not discussed it any meaningful ways to change. We each had our separate views. And now I would be gone for nearly seven months and thousands of miles away. We had each successfully set it aside. Life in the Army can be defined by extremes as well as norms, and this was an extreme time. We tuck away the weekends, the vacations, the time away from family, and rationalize that we will do something about it in the future. We further tell ourselves that the duty demands it, and we are all usually correct in all of this rationalization. Although correct, we are not necessarily right. I always envied the people whose lives seemed to conform so well so much on schedule in accordance with the next move, the next Army operation. The next case of cancer?

Many myths bind us. So many times we learn to stay behind the facade that we construct so well around our work. But sometimes the defenses all come down and we see ourselves without the symbols and decorations of the rank and the job and without the picture perfect family relationships, and we stand naked before who we are. Such was a moment on the beach and such was the first moment in a long time between Debra and I, without pretenses and symbols. We had only each other and we knew it, but we also knew that we would have to hold the thoughts privately while once again apart.

"Mark, Why are you so closed about the cancer? Don't you trust me enough to tell me what hurts?"

"I don't know. I do love you. I just I think it's over and there is no use discussing it."

That small tumor had invaded my wife's life as well as my own, but we never discussed it as ours, only as mine. I had my demons, and she had hers. Despite the dramatic storm on the coast, the demons were to remain separate for some time to come. The wind drove us inside and suddenly there was nothing left to say.

As April approached, I knew that Debra was watching the calendar click off the days. When we were engaged ten years before this trip, we were separated by a thousand miles as we awaited her college graduation. Though we might have expected to grow used to separations, it is a part of Army life that is much like moving: more and more practice at the task does not make it any easier. Each trip becomes more, not less, difficult, and each passing week punctuated the time until my departure. In this nomadic life that prevents us from investing too much memory into home towns or schools or geographic connections, in this life that teaches us that places in and of themselves do not matter too much, we grow to value the people we love and the people we meet, not especially the locations.

The weeks passed rapidly. Leaving with an advanced party of staff and soldiers, I went to the Sinai and returned almost as suddenly. Then we were running the remainder of the deployment from Fort Lewis. Soon enough, the real departure date came. The picture of Jeffrey, then five years old, is burned into my memory. He tries to say good bye, but can only cry. When I came home after my brief trip, in the magical world of a five-year-old child, he gleaned that Daddy was home. The idea that Debra was taking him to the base to see me mean only that we were going to see airplanes, not that I was leaving again.

I was at the hangar for a few hours before she met me there with both boys. Distracted with a few last minute details, like always, I could not give them the attention I wanted to give them and that they deserved. I was not very good at giving much of myself back then in any scenario, and certainly not in those where I was sad.

Sean was eight years old and absorbed the entire scene. He soaked it in. Not only the company formations in colorful berets and desert camouflage uniforms, not only the bands and the music, but also the small things; the hugs good bye, the looks of love and parting. Like many other times in his short life, he would mature in moments, not months or years. I have always seen him much like I see myself relative to how time passes and how time affects. We may suffer along and gain no benefit whatsoever from experience, and miss in championship form the point of the day. But at the strangest and most unexpected of times the lights will come on and we become complete sponges, synthesizing things that we do not even realize we have comprehended, some time in the past. My older son has had this gift, it seemed to me since the time of his infancy. My wife and I have frequently noted late at night in the tiny hours of the morning, how he made it through his first day. The day that also began in Tacoma, Washington, where he was born in the hospital where I was treated for cancer some nine years later. The temperature in Tacoma, Washington on that July day in 1978 was an unheard of 99 degrees, and at 8:00 PM it had relented not one degree as my wife burst small blood vessels in her face and chest trying to push him out into our world. Sean Gerner left his mother's womb reluctantly, asleep from the effects of the drugs and not yet ready to work his lungs in the world. An APGAR score of one, then two, on a scale that demands at least six or seven for survival and nine for health was not the best of signs for our first child. His first minutes were somewhat prophetic of his years that would follow. Although his childhood years were spent mostly on military posts, and the codes of behavior tended to follow stark lines with clean borders, Sean learned early on about the shades and tinctures of life.

His eight scant years were enough to teach him his father was going away for a purpose, but also that the purpose did not balance out the fact that I would leave behind something that I both needed and that I would have a hard time retrieving upon my return.

He pulled himself through birth with the help of a spirit or an angel, or something, and ever since he showed qualities that are unique in children. Sean showed great strength form the moment he was born, not two miles distant from this spot on the ground he was in another moment, one more in several to be in his next still very few years.

Until he actually saw the C141 transport aircraft in the hangar, five-year-old Jeffrey had not sense of my impending departure. After I checked the final manifest and did the small formation for the last of the soldiers that made up the final group to go, I just turned toward Debra, Sean, and Jeffrey and I waved and walked onto the plane. There was no more talking. When he finally realized what was happening, he began to cry and could not stop all night, cried himself to sleep.

Forty hours later we were at the airstrip at the town of Sharm El Sheik, in the southern tip of the Sinai, part of the land that Israel turned back to Egypt as part of the peace agreement in 1981.

The soldiers' routines developed quickly and we followed our well laid out plans. Time for them on the outposts over the two hundred mile border was challenging and isolated, but the weeks that followed a rotation on duty with some rare opportunities: tours in Jerusalem, in Cairo, and in Mount Sinai, for example. Altogether, the six months were much like duty for soldiers everywhere, especially on these kind of operations. Long periods of boredom and routine punctuated by surprises and excitement. Our excitements tended to group around the medical evacuation of civilian tourist. The occasional posturing of either the Israeli or Egyptian side had surprisingly little impact on what our soldiers did or how we lived. Long periods of routine accented by the occasional punctuation of excitement. It was, in the purest form, soldiering. A real mission, an important one, and one that offered the chance for camaraderie without the traditional requisite enemy to lend focus. We were doing well.

The desert's night was immensely quiet, as if to tell me how ancient and powerful it was. I was deep in sand, deep in the night, seeking out my direction on this nighttime compass course as part of the Infantry test I promised I would pass while here. I watched all of them; the dippers, the planets, and my all time favorite, Orion, the hunter. His figure spans a chunk of the sky and his the center star in his waist belt is Rigoula. To naked eyes from earth, this star appears to be the center of a clearly balanced and symmetrical formation. Three stars in the belt, with distinct and linear arms and legs that emit from the torsoe, and the arch of the bow that cirlces around the broad shoulders of a strong male figure. Or so it appears. In fact the stars are millions of light years apart, and the Orion nebula's mystery is only partially unlocked by the Hubbell telescope. Its form covers distances of the galaxy so vast they border on the philosophical. But on this night, his eyes seemed to focus not on the bear Ursa Major, the Big Dipper, but rather on me. The sand and the earlier scirroco winds mixed new scents in my nostrils.

The multitude of stories across the centuries that this land held. Tribes both ancient and modern crossed the land. In was in search of eight compass points on the ground on a land navigation course, the shifting sand and the lack of features were not my difficulties. Normally, my pace at night at Fort Lewis was one hundred and five paces for each one hundred meters of distance, through the woods and broken terrain. By contrast, here in the sand, it took one hundred and twenty paces in the day and one hundred eighty at night to cover the same distance. It takes some practice to find the points that were each some four hundred to six hundred meters apart on various directions. So my focus was on the problems at hand. Constantly counting paces to measure distance and checking my direction against the compass azimuth, I had great fun in completing the course even the practice courses, each night, on my own. In two more nights, this would be done.

Two mornings later, with the clock showing four A.M., I slowly warmed under the weight of the pack and my hands tensed around stock of the M16A1 rifle. The end point of my twelve-mile march is in sight almost immediately as I begin on a course that takes me past a Bedouin camp and camels, all hobbled with ropes to show claim. No camels are wild here any more. They are all owned by some one. I was strong, healthy and I was about to conclude this event in record time, at least for me. "There is no cancer left in me," I remember silently convincing myself. This final walk would expel the demons for good. The cancer simply had no place in a life and a body that could do this.

But in June that began to change. I needed to go for the medical tests. The July day began in its usual way. I awoke at 4:30 so that I could run in the somewhat cool air before dawn. The sun rose dramatically over the Red Sea as I finished my third run of the camp's perimeter wire. It would be a hot one, even by the standards of the southern Sinai in July. The lifeguard crew entered the Red Sea to begin their morning workouts in some of the most beautiful water in the world. This place that held such history and held millions of stories was where I became truly interested in one story, mine.

I considered the route: north to the Dead Sea, then west to Jerusalem for one night, then on to Herzlia on the Mediterranean coast. My breathing was suddenly erratic and I was sweating. There was a sharp pain in the pit of my stomach. There was another pain where the surgery had been and I wondered what was happening to me, as if the surgery were again happening. It was the briefest of moments, but also the most unmistakable: it was there. The cancer that fit so neatly into my life because it had gone as quickly as it came, was now intruding.

We stopped at "Checkpoint Three Alpha," on the coast of the Red Sea, with Jordan across the way. The sergeant in charge of the squad was a man I knew quite well. I liked him.

"How are you, Sergeant Gonzalez?"

"Fine, sir. The troops are doing fine, sir, better than I expected" He had the soft-spoken modesty of a strong man and a caring leader. It was no coincidence that his soldiers had such high morale. He was a "pro" in every sense of the word.

We talked for a while about the usual: water, hygiene, food, medical needs, any problems he might be having. The routine kind of questions that always yield some very non-routine responses.

"We're fine, sir. Maybe some checking again on why the mail was so late. Despite what the admin folks say, we are not getting mail until a week after it gets into the country. As far as other things, the chow. Can someone get us more fresh vegetables?" Small things are the most important to soldiers, and I promised I would again work on them. We each shared a laugh and as I turned to go, he asked, "Hey, Major Gerner, aren't you happy that "EIB" is done? All my men got it. It was good to see you there."

We crossed the border into Israel and drove first to Tel Aviv, then along the Mediterranean coastal highway to Herzlia. The people at the small medical center expected me and blood tests and the CAT scan were all prepared. I met with a pleasant woman, the staff urologist who was educated at Duke University and then served in the Israeli Army. She chatted for a while about the Sinai and how most people in Israel appreciated American soldiers who came there for peacekeeping. Suddenly, though, she stopped talking and began to concentrate on the

films. No more than a moment, a few seconds, really, and again I
was in trouble, totally under the control of her next order.

"I am concerned that there may be a spot on your liver. Here,
see, I'll show it to you." She pointed to some obtuse form that
looked something like a cigar. I was still getting used to the
view. The films are taken as if looking down through the top of
the head, and they take pictures every five centimeters. The films
depict spots, showing the density of what might be growths. I
saw a tiny white dot on the cigar, and I agreed that it might be a
big problem, but I had no idea what she meant.

"See this? This spot is what bothers me. True, it is very
small, but I still do not like it."

"I can't say I'm crazy about it either. What do you want to
do?" I had already resigned myself to the fact that whatever I
said, the doctors would be in charge again anyway, so I may as
well just listen to her.

"I want to do a liver function test. It will take some time and
be quite uncomfortable, but in your case it is worth it."

I did not even want to ask what it meant. The more she
talked, the more upset I became. So now someone another doctor
thinks I need another test. I was wondering in what century this
test was developed and what they would do to me. All I could
remember was the lymphnagiagram when they wanted my feet
sliced open in order to find, good point, to find what? I had
forgotten. Now she wanted to do something to my liver. What in
the world would this be?"

She called Doctor Fox in Tacoma, then a consultant back at
Duke. After a while, she told me that the test was really not
necessary after all, that the spot on the film seemed to be a part
of the permanent makeup of my liver, and that apparently it
shows up on every CT scan I have had, so she assumed then that
there was nothing abnormal about the scan. She told me there
was very little likelihood that anything was wrong, and even if

there was, they would "catch it" upon my scheduled six-month examination once I went home. She emphasized once again the importance of the periodic blood tests, x-rays, and CT scans, and told me not to worry. As a matter of fact, she explained, the frequency of the tests I was getting would be sure to find anything before it grew. In Israel, for example, most doctors would not prescribe such aggressive testing after testicular cancer. They would simply wait and see if anything developed again. I thanked her, promised to take her advice, and checked my watch. Ten minutes had passed from the time she noticed the spot until the moment we parted.

The visit was once again "routine." It was another of my momentary looks into the processes, the vagaries and interpretations of how cancer patients are tested and evaluated, the emotional roller coaster rides. I have frequently re-lived every detail of this trip to the Medical Center. Each image, each spoken word, remains crystallized in my memory many nights have found me crying out and then remaining awake to ponder the details of this trip to the small hospital on the Mediterranean coast. How would I ever be able to handle this? How could I go on? Was all of this pain and trouble and fear and doubt something that was a part of my character somehow?

Without knowing it, I had joined a club of extraordinary people who survive cancer. We react on visceral levels to medical appointments. We know a great deal of detail about ourselves. We reluctantly give up untold pieces of privacy and allow countless strangers to touch, poke, and prod. Some of the small prices of recovery. Any test can change quickly to more surgery, treatment, and something worse. Any test can be the first step on another narrow hard road of pain, fear, of treatments and surgery. Every cancer test is pregnant with something.

After Herzlia, I drove south toward the Dead Sea to camp at the base of Masada. The path to the top of Masada begins at the lowest point ever surveyed on the planet, some 960 feet below sea level. The climb to the top of the large plateau ends at sea level, one of the ironies of geography in a part of the world where there are many such ironies. Aromas mixed in the pre-dawn cold of the air; the flowers and milk weed foliage from the trail and salt from the Dead Sea combined into a kind of natural perfume that intoxicated the senses. There were shadows of rocks in the silent, crimson light. The quiet trail was leading me to new places.

In the year 66 CE a group from the Zealot tribe captured Masada from the Romans. King Herod had built a great fortress here from which he envisioned defending himself both from the tribes and from Cleopatra of Egypt. The Zealots' taking of the fortress is largely held as the beginning of the revolt, or the "Jewish War" a book by Josephus ben Matitiahu, later known as Josephus Flavius when he joined the Roman legions. Four years later, in 70 CE, the revolt ended in Jerusalem, thirty miles away. But in Masada, the Zealots held on for two more years and did so until the procurator Silva invested the fortress in 72 C.E. When he arrived at Masada, Silva found the band of Zealots were ready to fight, and had no mind to retreat or surrender, even in the face of his Tenth Legion, a force that numbered somewhere between ten and fifteen thousand soldiers. The Romans built eight camps to surrounding the 967 men, women, and children on Masada, but the fortress stood for some months before the tragic ending. Josephus Flavius recorded El'azar's appeal to his people. According the to Josephus, El'azar's oration spoke in part,

> *...that will mean the end of everything if we fall alive into the hands of the Romans. For we were the first of all to revolt, and shall be the last to break off the struggle. And I think it is God who has given us this privilege that we can*

die nobly and as free men, unlike others who were
unexpectedly defeated.

The climax was not surrender, but mass suicide. After climbing for an hour, I sat and awaited the sun and I wondered how they did that, how they found the collective courage of their belief in their freedom. Looking on the amazing construction, the walls, the cisterns, the homes I thought about how timeless it was that this place was as lonely as it was fortified. Why did this spot suddenly become so personal?

Come on, get over this. There is nothing wrong with you
anymore. They got it all and you know that. It is just your
imagination. You're just a little tired. In this place where the
story of life and death is so vividly evoked. It was a
crossroads for me, a place and a moment when the
philosophical ideas connect with the physical realties in life.
Maybe we do all carry the seeds of our destruction.

Maybe patients enter into relationships with their disease and thereby discover themselves in new ways. I know that is what it did to me and I know it began at this time. I thought of myself as the classic fighter. The boxing skills practiced in earlier times were still a part of my self image and though they were a source of some pride, I wondered if they were beginning to hurt, rather than help me, especially in my struggle for a view of my recovery. Was I investing too much of a human character in the cancer when I considered it a boxing opponent? It was, after all, just a mass of cells. Simply because I could relate to boxing did not mean it would serve me in this kind of a fight. I knew this last point very well intellectually, but I could take an active role in no other way but to try to fight it toe to toe.

Herb was the recreational director for the camp, and began each day with either a bicycle ride or a swim and a song. He sang to whomever was there. He would greet all with a song. Maybe a shell he had picked from a snorkel adventure. And a story. On one of my morning runs, he told me how one day when he was feeding the fish while snorkeling something very big swallowed the pocket to his swim suit and towed him out about a mile from shore, and the only way to survive was to cut himself out of the suit and swim away naked.

I knew, everyone there knew, that Herb had been a prisoner of war. The higher headquarters of the MFO requested clarification on his record, partly because the US Secretary of Defense was to visit soon and the POW Medal was to be awarded to all who earned it. In the query, they asked me if Herb had been a POW in one war or in two. I told them I would find out. This came to be a little more difficult than it first appeared. Herb's wife was visiting him for a few weeks in camp; and on a Sunday morning, the three of us had one of those remarkable conversations not easily forgotten. It went something like this.

"Korea. Yes, yes," he answered in his New England accent. "I was a POW in Korea. I remember I came back across that bridge. I remember I was a prisoner in Korea. Now Vietnam, I don't remember that so well. Maybe I wasn't a POW there. We were always running away after our missions in the Special Forces." His wife broke in and asked a question that would appear absolutely crazy.

"Well Herb, if you weren't a POW, then why didn't I ever hear from you?"

"Well, I don't know. Maybe we were POW's, and maybe we were just lost," Herb answered.

I could see that if one of was crazy, they were crazy together, and it didn't matter much. What mattered was they remained together over thirty years, in the face of long separations, wars, even this confused state that the POW question triggered. They just sat and smiled and drank their coffee together, he trying to puzzle it out, she humoring and teasing, but also loving him.

Herb was a kind of prophet who did not speak of religion, a kind of healer who did not speak of medicine. His pain was in a broken relationship with a son, not in some vague and now forgotten prison camp. His life in the Sinai suggested that he was transformed. At about the time we prepared to return, my name was published on the Army's promotion list to lieutenant colonel, quite a surprise because it was a year earlier than expected. When the plane landed back at McChord Air Force Base in Tacoma, the first thing that struck me was how beautiful Debra looked. I knew I was home when I saw her eyes. If the eyes are windows to the soul, then we have touched each other's souls in many ways over the years.

"You're tired," was all she said. I smiled and answered, "Not that tired." I did not even realize that the boys were not there. We were about to speak again when the band's rendition of a Souza march song interrupted. We both smiled and then it was time to get on the busses and the cars to go to the battalion area. Turn in the weapons, account for all the equipment and the people, and then go home. We took an easy slow ride through the back way to the post toward our home in Spanaway. The scent of fresh pine washed over me. The deep greens in the fading sunlight of late afternoon seemed to flow into my very core. I had missed this place, and I was not prepared for the stark contrasts between my temporary home in Egypt and what I now saw and sensed.

It was my favorite time of year in one of my favorite places, and cancer was the last thing on my mind. Debra and I were convinced that the recovery was real and was permanent. I was healthy in every way, especially statistically. I was to be a "special projects officer" for the commanding general of he corps. So I departed the battalion, reluctantly, for more staff time. November brought a cold front that held snow, and I packed my skis and found my way to the mountain. I headed for Reflection Lakes in Mount Rainier National Park to fill a growing need to be alone. Fall does not keep for many weeks there and the summer is deceptively warm at the lower elevations, while the weather at elevations about 8,000 feet takes on winter chills very quickly. The elevation and the confluence of glaciers make some dramatic weather on the mountain. I found the lakes freshly frozen and the long paths through the woods all around them covered in powdered snow; I skied all day, alone.

Winter came quickly and I absorbed the new job. Debra and the boys and I spent most weekends involve in some family activity; we skied, fished, or just went to some attraction in the area. Debra and I went out to dinner to celebrate Valentine's Day, but we were both on edge. Without speaking, we each sensed what was wrong. The cancer had invaded the evening. Without thinking about it, I had selected the same place we dined on the Valentine's day two years earlier, just a week prior to my surprise entrance into the hospital.

Debra probed gently, "Mark, when do you see the doctor for your two-year checkup?"

I had not told her. I kept the appointment and this sort of business to myself. Besides, it was just a formality. The cancer was gone. I really didn't need the appointment to affirm this.

I casually answered with one word, "Tomorrow."

There was a pregnant moment of silence, when I did not know whether I had angered her or whether she agreed that the entire matter was routine.

Then, I experienced the terrible moment when she repeats the word I have just said. I know that whenever that happens, watch out. "Tomorrow?" she said with irritation and inflection that only she can express in a single word.

Then she said it again. One word "Really?" with the inflection and the expression in both voice and face that only Debra can deliver. The tone that accompanies one word to tell you that not only have you screwed up, but that she has your number from top to bottom, and you have only fooled yourself if you think you were being smart by hiding something. A lot of wives and mothers attempt this means of communication; Debra has mastered it.

"Yes, really," I repeated, in a tone that revealed I was caught in a bad mistake and that I was sorry. And that I loved her, despite my poor judgment. This was new to me, and I knew deep down that I was not handling it very well. I had just completed so many things that validated I was completely healthy. I simply did not want any energy going into cancer, and I did not want to discuss this.

She sensed this in me and her tone changed from one of characteristic cross-examination to one of trust and accommodation. She answered, "Well, I'm glad. He will clear you and it will be over."

She did not chastise me for excluding her. Instead, she provided one of those surprises that only she could. In a moment, the smoldering, growing electrical charge in the air between us was gone. Her beautiful eyes returned to their familiar deep beauty from the fiery daggers of the grand inquisitor I saw a few minutes earlier. She has always had the incredible ability to do that. If I wanted to be alone with my tests and my doctors, that was fine with her. It was not that I wanted to exclude her from this. It was simply that I saw no need to rely on her and risk her in what was going to be a very routine part of a now historical case of a mild form of cancer. Allowing me the luxury of going to the doctor in my own way. And her eyes told me so.

I mumbled to my salad that I forgot to tell her about the appointment. It was more a quibble than a lie, because I intended to tell her about it when it was done. I wanted to come home into one of those romantic movie scenes when the stoic husband quietly battles his own fight with some crisis, and heroically suffers through this private fight alone. I would give them the gory details when I was the danger had passed. I wanted to spare her, and by extension me, the reminders of the prospects of more disease. But under the spell of her lovely eyes and her knowing expressions, I failed miserably.

I expected the examination the next morning to find me free of cancer, and all of it would be behind me, a distant memory, and the demons that fill each of us would remain forever locked up. At some point in the evening, Debra and I silently agreed to drop the subject. The numbers were on my side, and that was all that mattered.

4 A NEW KIND OF FIGHT

The knot in my stomach started while I shaved. It grew
progressively tighter on the drive to the hospital. By the time I
arrived at the urology clinic, it was a sharp, stabbing pain.
Pictures of surgery replayed in my mind's eye and the nerve
endings in my lower abdomen felt the cuts, even though the
surgery was two years earlier. Days of radiation sickness were
again there in front of me. Odors like burning plastic, synthetic
and ugly, invaded my senses, and I could barely keep down
breakfast.

I put this aside, collected myself, and said hello to Doctor
John Vaccaro. We talked a bit about how I was doing, about how
I felt. Each of us believing in our own separate yet shared ways
that the cancer was gone, our talk was comfortable and casual.
We took some comfort not only in the general statistics, but also
in the belief that I had now earned entry into the statistical group
labeled free of disease and soon to be labeled recovered or cured.
John had the view of the surgeon; he knew the signs, the effects,
all the probable outcomes, and he had every reason to be
optimistic. This would be a "classic case" of taking the right
steps for testicular cancer and solving it. I had passed two years
and the prescribed treatment of radiation had obviously done its
job. I had the view of the patient. I wanted it to be over, and I

had every reason to think that was the case. I was finished with it. My only involvement had been to agree to the radiation and then to check in for blood tests and x-rays every three months. I had been the "good soldier" with all of that. Neither one of us really understood nor even realized the other's outlook, but we agreed on this point: a border between this case of cancer and the rest of my life was about to be crossed, and we each believed the new territory held the promise of health. We were each wrong.

His hands, tools strong and skilled, moved with precision. They began to palpate the remaining testicle. He stopped suddenly. I froze.

"Mark, can you feel this?" he asked. "It's small, very small, like a piece of sand, here, I'll find it again."

I told him I felt nothing. What I really felt was a weakened stomach, a cold sweat on the back of my neck, and the all too familiar tightening, the first signs of anxiety. My hands and feet feel as though they have been plunged into ice water. I could no longer hear his words for the thunder of the blood pumping in my ears. But I did not need to hear to know the words. I had another tumor.

Such were my first steps on a journey that I again could not control. Control the trip or not, it had begun and I was on my way to somewhere. I envisioned major surgery, had the sinking feeling that I was now in a war, and a war I had stumbled into without the right weapons or training. It is a well worn expression that the first victim in any war is the truth, and I determined right from the beginning of this one the truth would not evade me, and if the truth were to work against me, then I would do whatever it took to change it, to change the conditions of my sickness, of my life if necessary to beat this again. That was a lot of thinking for a few moments of time in the car, but for me time was no longer measured in minutes or hours, but in moments.

I already missed the simple things I knew would soon be denied me; playing ball with my kids, like taking a healthy walk with my wife, like going to dinner with good friends. Instead, my attention and time would go to treatments, waiting rooms, pills, painkillers, and endless speculation about my future; these would now be my constant companions, at least for a time. I knew that cancer had already won the round. The cancer had already fooled me into thinking that I was all right when the blood tests proved negative. It cheated, and it won the round.

"I will beat it," I told myself. 'I will learn to know it, then I will kill it." This time, I would learn to fight it on my own terms. This thought became my rope on a rock's slippery face. Somewhere in the background I heard the doctor's words faintly, as if from a far off place.

"I'll do surgery tomorrow. Tumors of the testicle usually do not spread from one side to the other, so maybe it is something else. But the only way to be sure is to take out the testicle and get a biopsy. If it is just some infection, then you will need to deal with the problems of no testicles. But you will know you will be free of cancer. If it is cancer, we'll decide what to do then."

There would be many more planning sessions, all of which were pointed, sharp, calculated, purposeful, and discreet. Each step was simple enough to understand, but taken together they form a chain that seemed to grow one complex puzzle from another. When the answer to a specific point was found, the meetings would abruptly end. The patient and the doctor both always want to believe that these decisions are part of some larger plan, some strategy, that will lead somewhere toward healing. But the reality makes that very difficult. I did not concern myself with the strategy; I was in the trenches, firing at the next target. If there was a strategy or a plan, it was not yet mine. I had no ownership of this disease, of this piece of sand in my one remaining testicle.

John said all of this in perfectly logical sequence. He began to paint for me a word picture of some geometric proof. The panic was slowly but relentlessly building as I heard bits and pieces of statistics of populations of patients, both living and dead. I did not want to hear any of this. I did not want to hear about statistical bases of any populations of recovered or sick patients. I had just learned that all of the averages now meant nothing to me. After all, I had gone from being ninety four per cent certain that I was healthy to a hundred per cent sure I was sick again, all in the matter of a doctor's examination. I was again being welcomed into a world where normal thinking and logic are turned upside down. A place where doctors and patients talk of how to cure the body by poisoning it. A place where information is held back because no one really knows how an individual patient will react to a particular treatment. The combinations are nearly infinite and all of it got down to how well I would decide to get.

I left the doctor's office. I did not know where to go. Turn left and go back to work or turn right and go home. I took a deep breath. The pine scented air again. I barely maintained my balance while I stumbled around the parking lot, looking for where I parked my beat up 1978 Volkswagen dasher. "This is 1989," I said out loud to myself. "Maybe it's time for a change." As I got into the old familiar car, I sought not newness, but familiarity of....of what?

The house would be empty. Debra was at work, teaching. Who should I tell first? What would I say? What mattered most? I turned right and drove toward home.

Five minutes later I stopped the car and stared out the window. I was in tears. Not from the pain or the fear that I felt now, but rather from the memory of the pain and the agony of what I remembered. Quite contrary to fearing the unknown, it was what I knew about cancer that I feared most. My problem was that I did know what it was.

To many people, the word "cancer" is still synonymous with death. The fear that it inspires cannot be ignored or set aside. Intellectually, everyone knows that they will die. Though I had just been through cancer, I was not prepared for what would happen next. I never considered death in personal terms until this moment. Yet the fear did not spring from the fear of death. It came instead from my difficulty in returning to the life of a cancer patient. My tears stopped. I got myself under control, drove to the house, and called my wife, and asked her to come home right away.

When Debra got home, she looked at me and sat down without saying anything.

"They found another tumor." The words drained all energy from me. Exhausted, I sat in stillness and detected a shock wave so strong in Debra that it was almost visible. The new hope we had found in recent months was replaced by the invasion of disease. Even before we knew the details, we both realized our lives had been thrown out of control once again.

But we could not yet face it. We talked around the facts of the news, not daring to touch on what it might mean. We began to measure our time not in units of the clock but instead in visits to various doctors. Debra began to talk quietly and continued for what seemed several minutes. She told me how she knew that I would be able to fight it again.

"Mark, you know you are very strong. You will beat this again."

"How do you know that?"

"I can't tell you how, other than I know you and I know this is not your time to go. You have too much to do for this to stop you. Too many people need you and I have faith that you will be here for it."

"Well, maybe, but I don't share that right now. If I have so much to do, then why do I need this? I don't know if I can beat this again. I don't really know how I beat it the first time."

"You have to pay more attention to yourself. I'll help you. Starting right now."

"I don't know that I can do it. I don't want that surgery and I don't want any radiation or chemotherapy. I'm so afraid it will just take everything out of me." Then, an added thought, "How is Sean going to take all of this again?"

Once again, my initial worries were about Debra and the kids, not about me. But this time my motive was not generosity, but a terribly cold fear that my very life was in danger, and I needed to shift the attention onto someone else, onto Sean. I grew wearier with every sentence. For now, there was nothing left to say.

The shock of this day stands apart from all others for me. It marks a great change in direction. In the minutes at the doctor's office, I moved from my old life to a new view of life, a new view of my disease. In the Sinai, I began to see myself differently, but did not yet know why. At this moment in time, while Debra and I talked over the reality of another bout with the disease, while we considered how my life, our lives would be yet again transformed in ways we could not know, while all this happened, my life changed. I had entered again the world of cancer, again, a world where all my energy would have to be directed at survival while all notions of pleasure, or growth, or anything else I valued would again be on hold, or so I thought.

I have known my limits before, but I could not estimate the extent of the suffering to come. The medical reasons for my returned disease did not matter. I asked myself the "Why me?" question only once, then never allowed it again. Images of career, future plans, my family, and every other consideration all became very much secondary to cancer. I began to consider the disease of mine, and I knew I would need to find my connections within it. Before, it was the property of the medical profession, of the systems around me that I had to accept. But cancer was now mine.

Even though the prospect of another operation loomed large, I took some comfort in the knowledge that it would be the same operation as two years earlier. Doctor Bill Fox would remove the testicle using the same kind of cut he used before on the other one. "At least now I'll be balanced again," I joked with him. He would then evaluate the biopsy, decide what it was, then make a plan. For now, whatever complications might arise from being without testicles were minor concerns when measured against what had to be done. The process began as if it were the first time and I was in the same terrible position as before, feeling helpless and without words as friends and visitors came and went. I began to think that maybe they would find that the piece of sand was actually some infection, and this would all be worry over nothing.

But that was wishful thinking. The operation was relatively easy. It had very little physical pain. The doctors knew from the texture of the tumor that it was some kind of cancer. They would not make a judgment until the biopsy. Once again, the waiting. When the biopsy returned a week later, doctors Fox, Vaccaro, and Debra and I met. They told us the cell was embryanal carcinoma, and then they began to explain.

"This is an aggressive cell," Vaccaro said.

He looked at me for a moment, as if he wanted those words to sink in before continuing. But "aggressive cell" could not sink into my brain because it is one of those code words in the language of cancer. The term has no meaning or confused meanings until you learn the code. The doctor thought he said something I should understand, but the only message for me was confusion.

"What do you mean by that?"

"The cell you had two years ago was seminoma. That cell responds to radiation treatment, it usually is killed by the levels of radiation we gave you."

Again, he looked at me for a long moment before he said, "Mark, we don't really know what happened. It is very unlikely that testicular cancer spreads from one side to the other. If it begins to metastasize or to spread, it goes up the lymph systems. That's why we have had you on this regime of the chest x rays and the CT scans."

The idea that this was a new cell meant that the carcinoma was either present two years and not detected, or that this was a new case. This presented a problem. The cancers are different in character and carcinoma does not die under radiation. There was discussion of whether I wanted a prosthesis for the testicle. This seemed to be a rather important to them, and I just looked at them like they were from Mars. They had just told me that cancer was back, that they would need another biopsy, and no one really knew yet what would happen next. Now they want to know how I would feel about appearances. I simply did not know nor did I care very much about what it would look like. The idea of how I might feel changed in that way was silly to me. Within these "routine" decisions, the traumatic and the practical parts of life intersect. Small details such as "do you want a prosthesis?" I learned to understand that they were simply trying to do their jobs efficiently. It came down to the practical matter of "why open him up twice when we can do both jobs at once." I agreed to the prosthesis.

John continued to describe the cell. He said it was "embryanal carcinoma," a very aggressive cell. The "embrayanal" part meant that that it was still in its embryonic, or early stages. But when it moves, it does so very quickly through the lymphatic system, and even in its earliest stages it is very aggressive. So the doctors had to act quickly but they simply did not yet know the best strategy. They had to consult with a number of other doctors first, to get a best judgment.

Then he added another point, "We have to begin the process of a medical board. We will probably process you out of the Army."

Debra changed. She sat up in her chair. Her face went from pleasant and cooperative to challenging and assertive. Her tone became sharp. Her instincts told her that this was going to be a great adventure in pain and difficulty for me, and she was not about to sit still and listen to something about this now, not without proof.

"Why does he have to have another medical board," she asked.

"Well, it will be a second case of cancer, and we will take out the remaining testicle. It's one of the conditions that means a soldier must leave the Army," one of them said.

"How do you know that? Why are you so sure he will need to leave? What if he gets better?" she fired back in rapid response.

They checked the regulations and to their surprise, she was right. There was no need to start any board. Not on the basis of losing a testicle, anyway. My, our, first small victory. The focus then shifted to the operation and me.

It was the briefest and most important of exchanges. I had never seen my wife quite like that before. I always knew she loved me, but never before saw her as my advocate. There was real power in her when she mustered herself to my defense. How easily she challenged not the doctors, but the idea that in my time of pain and weakness, someone was about to begin a process that would take something away from me, my profession. All of us, to include the doctors, learned a lesson from Debra that morning.

John's intent to "act "quickly" was an understatement. Three
days after our talk, he called and asked us to come back and
review the next steps. He had consulted with many physicians,
and he recommended further surgery, extensive surgery,
followed by in patient intense chemotherapy treatments. The
surgery is known as "lymph node resection," meaning the
removal of all lymph nodes in the chest and abdominal area. The
lymphatic system is made up of hundreds of nodes distributed
throughout the body. The objection of the operation was to
remove about sixty such nodes in the areas of the chest and
abdomen. The principle behind the operation is similar to certain
infantry tactics. If looking for an enemy, one way is to take away
all the places he may hide. Give the enemy no means to rest or to
supply, and over time, the enemy will lose. When it comes to
battles, it is usually far better to win than it is to find a way for
the enemy to lose by his own hand. And this is where I had to go
to work and think not only about how the doctors were going to
force the cancer to lose. But how would I win? The tactical idea
was simple enough, but without a personal strategy I could lose
nonetheless.

As advanced as medicine has become, the treatments for
cancer remain heavily weighted toward only the physical aspects
of the cells and the things that generally poison them, and it
remains combinations of surgery, radiation and chemotherapy.
So there was no talk yet of what would happen after the surgery.
That would have to wait until they did biopsies on the nodes they
would remove.

The doctors again let this sink in and they watched my
reactions closely. The surgery was a major undertaking. Internal
organs would all be removed, nodes removed, and then repaired
and returned. The plan was to take out all nodes of the lymph
system and then microscopically evaluate what was removed.
The operation was expected to take about six hours, with four

surgeons. But perhaps the most difficult part was the way in which they would render the judgments over what would happen throughout the operation and after.

Nothing showed on the routine tests, meaning that the level of cells in my system did not register, even though they had massed into a small tumor. We would all hope that the grain of sand was the extent of the problem. The blood tests, CT scan, and x-rays would somehow confirm that this was all that was amiss. In other words, I could take a "wait and see" strategy once the lymph nodes were out. But the problem with the wait and see plan was that it had just failed. None of these tests had indicated that the cancer returned. Only the doctor's physical exam told me that.

This was to have been the last examination. That was why Deb and I were upset the night before. We were upset over the anticipation. Now we had something real to be upset over. The doctors did not know how to act when they determined that it was another tumor. Not only was I going to "make it" through cancer, I was one of their star patients. I was still on active duty. I was returned to full duty, and obviously doing quite well with the announcement of my promotion. The goal of the Army's medical department is not only to treat, but to get soldiers back to as close to full duty as possible, and I was great evidence of this. They were all pulling for me. They had come to know me and I could see that they were hurting in their own way as they advised me on what to do next.

A lymph node resection is a complex operation. The doctors had to coordinate moves and follow a detailed plan over the expected eight hours of surgery. They would leave behind a set of stainless steel clips to bind the wounds. The surgery would affect the penis area and the nerves around it. By avoiding some cuts in the area, the experienced urologists could allow me to retain all sensitivity in the area for sexual activity. With so many emotions at work, this was only a minor point, an insignificant detail. I was considering the potential spread of cancer, and I was not concerned with the physical aspects of how I would have sex in the future. But I managed to give it some attention and I told them clearly to do whatever it outlook to keep me intact as much as they could.

Bill Fox planned to open with a long incision up my center from the top of the penis to the base of the breastbone. When they clipped me back together, it took some forty-four staples. The plan was to remove all my intestines and then nurses would assist in holding the organs out over the table as the doctors would remove the nodes attached, and then sew parts of the intestines and clip other parts back together. They would then go after all of the other nodes in a very systematic way.

The set of nodes in the area of the penis presented some unique problems. The surgeon told me he could avoid the nodes around the penis so that he did not damage any of the nerve endings and maintain the normal sensations for sexual activity. But there was a risk in allowing any node to remain. After all, the entire point of the operation was to remove them. John said, "You're right, Mark, if we don't touch that node, then we do leave behind a place where the cells can grow. To be as safe as we can, we should take it out."

"OK, then let's take it out," I said.

"We will do it like this," he continued. He began speaking very logically, mechanically, and I was surprised by his approach. He may as well have been describing some procedure on a car. If this, then that, if that then this, in the now all too familiar talk of systems connected to systems, processes that fit into other processes. Intellectually, this should have assured me; he knew what he was saying. He knew how to do this. My reactions were visceral because it was one more thing I had to do, one more piece of information I did not want to absorb. I was

beginning to wonder if I would ever end this journey. A slow
burning panic began.

He started to draw some pictures. Explaining that the cuts
would alter the way things work, he was careful to tell me that
all sensations would be the same, but the way in which certain
familiar things flowed would be slightly altered. It even had a
name. Medical processes, especially ones like this, seem to
operate in code much of the time. The condensing of ideas into
forms of short hand and code that can misrepresent the physical
realities. Because the doctor and I knew each other well, I
insisted on a clearer explanation. He explained retrograde
ejaculation in layman's terms. The point of the operation, of
course, was to remove the lymph nodes and in order to take out
the node in the area of the penis, some nerves must be severed
and the canal is altered in order to attack the lymph node. But
removing the nodes in this area meant severing some nerve
endings that affected the function of the ejaculatory duct and the
urogenital diaphragm, and the bulbourethral or Cowper's Gland.
This meant that during ejaculation, the flow out through the
gland is diverted in another direction because the nerve no longer
holds a valve closed. The action is similar to that of a door that
swings open with the wind; one must apply force to hold it shut,
and in this case the force of the nerve would not longer be there
so the valve would be free to rotate. This would mean that
although the sensation would be the same, the flow would not
always be out the front, having been ciphered off in another
direction. Hence the term "retrograde ejaculation."

If I were going to save any of these nodes for any reason at
all, including how I ejaculated, then why even do this
enormously complex and clearly painful operation. Why not
simply do what the doctor in Israel described? Just take the "wait
and see" approach, and set aside the operation. For all its

precision, it remained a blunt instrument. I decided to take all the nodes; all the places the disease might grow.

On the day I checked in and underwent preparations, a very unusual snowstorm brewed. By nightfall, snow was falling in record levels, and the road conditions allowed no one to drive to see me. Mount Rainier, a place with some of the deepest snowfalls in the world was only thirty miles distant, yet never a flake drops here in town, only rain. I dutifully drank the barium sulfate to empty the bowels. One of the first of my many sleepless nights.

My breathing became slow and deliberate. I felt much like when I was eighteen and nineteen years old and awaiting a boxing match at West Point. While training for each match, the drills and the contact seemed to make great sense. But in those terrible minutes before the bell, it made no sense at all and I would always resolve that this was the last bout. Fear, confidence, and doubt mixed together again. Would all the cuts go as planned? Would I awake with some surprise condition?

It is two in the morning and there is no chance of sleep. Rivers of emotions wash over me. Each feeling is distinct, but each is difficult. Images in my head depict pictures of both the future and the past. Scenes of baseball diamonds; athletic plays, swings of a bat, running hard with that mix of dust, freshly cut grass, and exhaust fumes that only a city park can offer. How old? Thirteen, sixteen? The hitting is clean, fast, and solid, so it must be later, it must be high school. Does the world await? I do not care. It is good enough to stay here. It is early spring. The warmth is new and the senses alive and connected to the muscles that suddenly find speed and fluid motion, encouraged by the sudden and surprise increase in air temperature around them. The day is only about baseball. There is no room for illness here, certainly no room for cancer.

Why the pictures? If I get the chance, what will I change?

The intravenous anesthesia starts to flow, sending me somewhere else, somewhere apart from this room. I hovered above myself and felt giddy, happy, and numb. Two very cheerful and very strong nurses spoke in friendly tones to me and then I was naked in the bed. Then a gown quickly moved over me and I was on my way. They slowly and cheerfully wheeled me down the corridor, while some familiar faces said some things I did not hear. Someone told a joke. Then they asked me to count backwards from ten. I got to seven when the lights went out.

Many months later, Debra told me that during the operation one of the nurses in the operating room would come to her throughout the operation and report the progress. The scenes were surreal, to stand powerless while someone described in detail how my intestines and lymph nodes were being dissected, then placed back together and re-inserted, all so that the surgeons could search of the disease. I understood the picture not only from her words, but somehow from a memory, as if I was recalling a scene that I witnessed. I had reconstructed the scene many times in my head.

"Your husband has surprised them," the nurse said with a small smile. I could picture the smile quite clearly, because Debra's face changed as she relayed the words of the surgical nurse. She smiled reflectively.

"He isn't bleeding at all," the nurse continued to Debra. "They have not given him any blood. That's a very good sign." Then came some of the details. She described how the surgeons had to move and hold parts of the intestines and other organs and how they worked together as a team through each step, carefully examining then removing the nodes.

This detail helped her get through the hours. Difficult as it is to visualize me in that condition, it would have been far worse to hear nothing or some sugar coated vagaries such as "I'm sure he'll be OK." The surgical team took some time to prepare, study and to practice. Surgeons who do this and procedures like this are among the most remarkable people. But they are only people, and from my experiences I have learned that they need thanks and credit and understanding much more than they get. The expectations we have out of surgeons such as my team are enormous. Probably far too great for the number of variables at work in this scenarios. But no matter the preparations, the operation takes on a kind of life of its own, and the team must assess as they progress. Any feedback at all helped her fill the terrible voids of time.

Some theories of pain postulate that the mind and the brain can recall every detail of every trauma to the body, even it the body was unconscious. There have been many times in the last five years when I recalled many specific moments of the surgery. I have felt the distinctions between small and large cuts. I feel the sense of fear and comfort both. The fear springs from the certain pain that awaits me. I flinch slightly with each move of the scalpel. But I take comfort in the idea that the unhealthy tissue and nodes will finally depart my body, giving it the chance to heal. I have had dreams of very specific voices and words that were exchanged in the operating room. Professional terms mixed with small talk. They were measures to relieve the terrible stress they feel if they allow themselves to consider the consequences of each cut and each judgment they make under hard, cramped, messy conditions. An excellent surgeon told me that the image is so different than the reality for him. He always feels like he is in the midst of a big mess, and he has to squeeze, poke, guess, curse, and search for things that simply do not come out easily. Blood and other organs get in the way, obscure his vision of the already difficult work. His plan remains etched in his brain, but distractions take him off the mark, and his mind's eye puzzles out the next moves, for the next moves are significant not only in relation to the plan, but also to how he assesses each discovery in this complex journey of surgery.

I wanted desperately to help in this, to help them make the puzzle a little easier, to do my part and somehow connect back to life, to discover a way through this new kind of fight. Old ways to battle enemies were not going to work. They were sufficient to survive, but not to live. My "wuzzes" were piling up in great numbers, and I had to work to appreciate a life without pain, maybe one must know and recall severe pain. I was fooled into the belief that it was all physical pain. Now in a new kind of fight, I could define neither the enemy nor the battle. The cancer had successfully hidden itself from me, even now that the tumor was out.

5 NUMB FINGERS AND LONG FALLS

Chemotherapy: Treatment of a disease with chemical substances.

The birth of modern chemotherapy is credited to the efforts of Paul Erlich in Germany during the early part of this century. While attempting to stain bacteria without staining the surrounding tissue, he speculated about some "magic bullet" that would selectively find and destroy pathogens but not harm the host. This idea provided the basis for chemotherapy, a term he coined.
--Microbiology, by Tortora, Funke and Case.

The cold began in my toes, rolled up the back of my legs and massed into what seemed a bag of ice at the base of my spine. My body was buoyed by lungs stretched to burst and it rose up through the cold, dark, lake trying desperately to escape the pain. My face broke the surface of the water and the harsh light of the recovery room ended the dream. I shivered to my core. Recovery rooms are frigid to control bleeding and shock. But it could not control my pain. As I realized where I was, a slow sickness

welled up. Metallic odors and tastes that mingled. I hardly
noticed the tubes stuck in my wrist, mouth, and my nose.
So cold. Why am I so cold?
The pain slowly but relentlessly cut through massive doses
of morphine. All my nerves were at its mercy. Somewhere in the
dim past of the last week were the surgeons' firm instructions to
begin to walk. I felt like each organ was being continually cut by
scalpels and when the orderlies lifted me onto the bed, all went
white. When I screamed, it was from deep within me; a sound I
had never before heard. I felt every part of every cut, and felt it
everywhere. I knew from the nurse's expression that something
was wrong.
"What's the matter?" I whispered.
She was a young lieutenant. She had eyes that told you
immediately that she was intelligent and caring, and that she was
eager to do well. But the sight of me shook her confidence.
"Nothing," she said quietly while she averted her eyes.
"...It's just that I did not expect..."
I decided to remove the pressure. I turned instead to Debra
and in her eyes I caught an image, the kind of picture I'd seen
only in nightmares. A strange mix of familiar and alien images
filled my brain. I was looking at a corpse of myself. Fear was
there. It was deep in a way that made it feel like it oozed in and
out of my soul. I wondered if I would ever again find myself in
the terrible image now in the mirror.
A device known called a "Nasogastric tube" ran from my
nose to my stomach. The tube is used to aspirate the contents of
the intestines. The idea is to prevent gas and fluids from
distending the coils of the intestines. The tube enhances the
process called decompression. The normal functioning of the
intestines, known as peristalsis, decreases or even stops for
twenty four to forty eight hours after an operation. The effects of
both anesthesia and the manipulation of the intestines (visceral

manipulation) impede the functions, so that tube is necessary to eliminate fluids, thus preventing vomiting, to relieve tension incision, and to aid the blood supply to the suture line, thereby providing nutrition.

It was important that the tube not come out of my nose. I found none of this particularly interesting until a nurse told me that if the tube came out, she would have to reinsert it through my nostril into my stomach. Her tone was so casual that the image of it did not even register. The picture of someone wrestling this thing down my nose and esophagus all the way to my stomach was nearly comical. The price of the sin of a sneeze.

Debra became my self-appointed "gate guard." She allowed no one to see me, to bother me, but especially for no one to gather some impression of me as hopeless based on my physical appearance. There was no strength in my voice, no glint in my eye, no energy for anything. Staples bound the wound up the center of my stomach and chest. My moans of pain were not to be heard by anyone but her. She determined that visitors could share some things with me, but not this. She did not want anyone to be frightened by me and thereby begin loose talk and rumor over my prognosis. She would allow only my closest of friends to be in the room with her.

Recalling the doctors' advice, and knowing that I had to do something very soon or I would fall victim to the ever increasingly complex process, on the third day I decided to walk. Debra helped me up out of bed. She held an arm around my waist. The hundred feet or so of hospital hallway began as therapy and turned into the longest march of my life. The goal was thirty feet. But two steps into the marathon, my legs and stomach locked up. The pain in my stomach built and my entire front felt like one tightened muscle. The incision cut me again with each step. Once again, nothing had prepared me for this. For reasons I came to understand much later, they omitted much of what lay ahead of me. But no matter their proficiency and compassion, no one could tell me what to do or how to feel, or how to get well.

Bill Fox told me that the intestines would take a long time to heal. He would not say how long and would not say what it would be like. He simply did not know. I wanted to go home. I wanted none of the painkillers, or anything connected to the hospital or the doctors. I felt I had somehow become responsible for this terribly frightening chapter of my life. If there was to be any good outcome of my cancer, then meant that I had to undergo the suffering alone. But it became too much, and Debra could stand it no more. She began to educate me. The only way for tissues to heal is for them to relax. She learned about the healing process within internal organs as patients recover from surgery, and she studied how nutrients are circulated and how the healing takes place. She related this to the instructions that the surgeons had given me and how the painkillers were in fact muscle relaxers and also neuro suppressers. No matter my dearly acquired vision of mental toughness, the fact remained that without the painkillers, the massive cuts would take much longer to heal. My body cried out to for relief. We sparred in the conversation that went her way.

"Mark, you have to take these."

"Why? I don't need them. I'll be fine without them. I don't want to get addicted to these medications. They're too strong. These are Tylenol three and that's just like codeine. I don't want them."

"You are going to take them. Stop giving me your "mental toughness crap" that you've fed to yourself for years. This isn't about how tough you are. It's about how stupid you are if you don't take them. And oh by the way, you can say you are tough, but it's me you'll be keeping awake all night with your crying in pain. Take them." I listened.

Only the natural recovery of the intestinal tissue could eliminate the air. The intestines would contract to push the air through the length of the thirty feet of the system, and as the air moved, much of the serpentine organ went into intense cramping. The cuts remained fresh within me and the pain remained sharp and biting, constant.

We waited for the results of the biopsies. The surgeons took samples from strategic nodes and tissue, looking for the cancer in its potential hiding places, and now they awaited the analyses. In almost military style, they use the biopsies along with other pieces of knowledge of the cancer to find out exactly where it is and then to predict its future movements. The idea is to attack at leas the immediate threat, and hopefully gain enough insight to devise an entire campaign. As for me, I was mentally moving more toward indirect methods to revisit my life, whatever the outcome of the next few days.

I had not yet met the people who occupy the oncology clinic, a place of great mystery and intrigue where it seems that architects of chemical equations consort with magicians to concoct potions. Helping them in their modern medieval tasks are all sorts of workers, sworn to secrecy as to what the "medicine" is and what it does. Without these loyal soldiers, the battle against cancer may go on, but the campaigns against patients would surely be in serious trouble. This one composed of oncologists and chemists is quite remarkable. It's team fights against a disease to save patients, and in the process it must figure out ways to work the poison with the patient in equations that must somehow balance. Most look to these teams for treatment and "cures," that warrant the miraculous, but produce only the mix of art and science called the practice of medicine. It remains a very dramatic, and a very sad, and a very ancient vocation, this search for how to treat the body so that it will rid itself of tumors and even cells that carry cancer.

When I agreed to enter into chemotherapy, I did not understand what it means. I considered only the data, the chances of cure. In a case like mine, where the disease returned in a new form and in a different testicle, that without some kind of intense chemotherapy, the chances of return again would be relatively high, something like six out of ten cases. I never found any statistics on such a scenario. But I trusted the anecdotal evidence that my excellent urologists related to me after they had done much consulting. I trusted my own strength to withstand the chemotherapy, even if it meant debilitating me to the extent that I may need to leave the Army, because the risk of not taking it might permit the carcinoma cells to spread rapidly. In cases of returned testicular cancer, chemotherapy cuts down the chances of recurrence to about only twenty per cent. In cases where the patients do not take the treatment, the recurrences can be as high as fifty per cent. Both of these numbers gave me some pause. I had joined the discreet population of the seriously ill, whose fates are measured in cold numbers. I was now a statistic. It was a relief to sign the form. Take every chance they give you, I told myself.

A week later I met the oncologist. As he spoke, it occurred to me that he could come to his conclusions about how to administer chemotherapy without even seeing me. The factors that go into such calculations are all about the chemical relationships between the tumor and the choices of drugs to administer to me. Cold as it may sound to the uninitiated, the patient, for a time at least, is only incidental to the process. I asked my friend Bill Fox about the idea. He said I was indeed correct, and then something I have tried to recall and hang on to through many challenges of healing. He said, "Doctors do not cure, do not heal. We merely set the conditions for the body and the person to cure themselves."

Chemotherapy has matured over time and its sophistication now allows prescriptions for either a substitution for or an addition to surgery. When added to surgery it goes by the term adjunct chemotherapy. But even now, there are no drugs that are truly selective for malignant cells. All chemical agents used in chemotherapy have some level of toxicity or poisonous effect on healthy tissues. Therefore, oncologists and the patients are presented with arrays of problems, some of which are about the kind of cancer cells and some of which are about the relationship of the drugs to healthy organs in the patient's body. Complex as it seems, in the end the plan will be based on the judgment of the doctors about how much punishment the patient can withstand. Though I found the doctors' concern for my future sincere, their focus was on strategies for "total cell kill," even if that meant some limitations for me.

Tumors that have a large growth fraction are susceptible to drugs that are known as **antineoplastic**, meaning the drugs work by slowing cell proliferation and division. The growth fraction means that a relatively large proportion of the cells in the tumor are engaged in cell division. Young tumors have a high growth fraction and are therefore more vulnerable to chemotherapy than are older tumors, which have simply been around a while longer and are less vulnerable to the killing effects of the chemical agents. I think chemotherapy goes beyond the art and the science of medicine and touches the borders of philosophy. It is a mix of the very direct weapons and the very indirect strategy. The chemicals in the arsenal of weapons are called antineoplastic (from the Greek anti + neos new, and plasma something formed). The term means a substance or a procedure that prevents the proliferation of malignant cells. Varieties of antineoplastic drugs, when used in combination and in sequence with other drugs, kill cancer cells. The regimes usually aim the drugs at identified targets, that is, cells that have a known form of development.

Some chemicals are **alkylating** agents, substances that contain alkyl radicals and therefore are capable of replacing free hydrogen atoms in an organic compound in the chemical reactions between agent and body. The point of these chemical reactions is to interfere with the mitosis and cell division of the cancerous cells. There are adverse effects of these antineoplastic drugs, determined by the same principles. Tissues of the body that have high rates of cell proliferation are the most susceptible to the toxic effects of the drugs. Normal tissues which have high rates of proliferation include the bone marrow, the hair follicles, the mucosal membranes of the alimentary tract, from the mouth to the rectum, making these areas particularly sensitive to the treatments. One effect is **leukopenia** (from the Greek for leukos + penes - poor). The term means an abnormal decrease in the number of white blood cells to fewer than 5,000 cells per cubic millimeter. The decrease may be caused by an adverse drug reaction or by radiation poisoning. Another condition is **alopecia** (from the Greek for *alopex*, fox or mange). It is a partial or complete lack of hair, resulting from age, endocrine disorder, or cancer treatment. A third effect is **ulcerative lesions**, crater like markings on the skin or the mucous membrane. These affects are common to all antineoplastic agents.

Anti cancer drugs are defined by the cycle of cell division for the kinds of cells they are designed to attack. Cell growth occurs in five phases: the resting state, the postmitotic gap, during which the building blocks of DNA are synthesized, the synthetic phase, during which the building blocks combine into DNA itself, the premitotic gap wherein the spindle, a form in the cell nucleus, is produced, and mitosis, or cell division. These stages of cell division are important because most antineoplastic drugs can act only on cells that are in a specific stage. Such drugs are known as **cell cycle specific**. Other agents, such as alkylating agents and cisplatin, by contrast, are cell cycle nonspecific, and can act on cells during any phase. Chemotherapy derives from objectives that are seldom achieved, yet always necessary. The stated objective in chemotherapy is the eradication of all malignant cells, known as **total cell kill**. Anything short of this is not considered a "cure" in clinical terms because a single surviving malignant cell can ultimately divide and grow and ultimately kill the host, the body. The body's immune system is not sufficiently reliable to defend against malignant cells because for the most part, tumor cells escape the notice of the system. Simply put, the body can easily be fooled into reading a tumor as healthy, as part of the system, and not as an invader.

Most tumors develop resistance to drugs. Tumor resistance can come in several forms, to include **cytokinetic resistance**, (cells are proliferating slowly), and **schedule resistance** (when the antineoplastic drugs' frequency is not correctly coordinated with the growth state of the tumor.) In the relationship of tumors to drugs, these are known as inherent characteristics, and then there are also kinds of resistance known as **acquired resistance**, biomedical changes that improve a cell's ability to withstand the action of a drug.

Before the plan was solidified, there were still more factors to consider. One of the most important was the bone marrow. Most of the drugs suppress the marrow, complicating the process because the agents vary in the extent to which they slow or stop the components of the marrow and the white blood cells. The primary function of white blood cells is to fight infection. They are produced in three-week cycles. Some of the main components of bone marrow are **granulocytes**, of which there are three: basophil, eosinophil, and neutrophil cells, and **thrombocytes**, platelets, which are disc-shaped, white blood cells. Platelets are the smallest of the cells of the blood. They contain no hemoglobin, and they are essential for blood coagulation. Added to this are the red blood cells, which carry oxygen, and **lymphocytes**. Lymphocytes comprise about twenty five per cent of the white blood count and are made up what are known as B cells and T cells. The function of the B cell is to search out, identify, and bind itself to specific antigens. Antigens are proteins that cause the formation of an antibody and react with that antibody. T cells are often called "killer cells," because they secrete chemical compounds that then react with B cells to destroy foreign bodies. Taken together, then, any attack on the functioning and growth of bone marrow is a serious blow to the body.

Bone marrow suppression varies in how rapidly it develops and in how long it persists. In my case, the plan was the "VBP" regime for disseminated testicular cancer." The code designates the combination of chemicals: "V" for vinblastin, "B" for bleomycin, a drug given for several weeks after the "in patient" portion of the sessions were completed. The "P" was for cisplatin, a derivative of platinum. Cisplatin is given some hours after the vinblastin. Each drug has its own protocol in combination with others to address the specific stages of cell development that the biopsy tells the oncologists to expect in the tumors. The carcinoma that my biopsy revealed is a cancer that invades tissues and establishes bases in the peripheral parts of tissues. It then moves from these foreign bases through the lymph system, and seeks out other tissues. When it moves, it does so rapidly. The biopsy on my tumor labeled it embryanal, meaning it is in the embryo, or in the early stages of its cellular development. In most dynamic relationships, timing matters, and it especially matters in chemotherapy. There is a relatively short window of opportunity for the treatment to produce its effects, and the time is connected to when the tumor is removed.

Muscle tissue does not long withstand the relentless assault of poisoned blood and tissue. The oncologist derives certain combinations of chemicals from lists according to the nature of the cancer cells identified in the pathology. The idea is to time the poisons entering the system so that they kill the cells. The prescription's paradox, however, lies in two major areas. Another piece of the puzzle is the measure of progress. As much as I wanted to believe that my body fought off the disease, the principle behind chemotherapy does not rely on a healthy body. Instead, the objective is to make the body uninhabitable for cancer cells by poisoning the lymphatic system. Eventually the body will recover, while the building blocks of tumors will not. "Progress" is measured in the white blood count; driving it down, putting the body into a weakened state. It works on the idea that we cannot measure what we want, the cell count of cancer. But we can measure the white blood count, and by extension, deduce something about the health of the tumor.

The oncologist establishes a base line from which the oncologist can measure the high and low points of the white blood count, or "wbc." Chemotherapy is usually begun when the wbc is close to its low point. Subsequent treatments begin when the wbc is once again at its trough, usually every three weeks. I had my own idealistic goals of rapid recovery and techniques of self reliance and visualization, but these ran smack into the cold realities of chemical relationships. There were few numbers that explain a case like mine. These recurrences are rarely fatal, but still they still present difficulties. Is the only measure of patients' recoveries the measure of survival?

To keep the patient alive while the oncologists poison the cancer, they "snow" the patient with other chemicals that balance out the poisoning affect of the lead and the platinum affects. Only by counting the white blood cells and showing a significant decrease could the oncologist get a hint about the effect of the formulas he came up for me. That is, we cannot measure the actual cancer cells or tumors when they are microscopic. But we can measure the white count, and we surmise that if white cells are dying off, then cells of cancer are also dying. We measure what we can.

I felt each drop of poison leave the bag of fluids and hit my arm through the tube. It began its movement warm, then turned very hot, and the heat moved relentlessly up my arm, immobilizing the entire side of my body. It rapidly progressed to the shoulders and the neck, and finally it engaged my head. I dreaded how my stomach would react. It was filled with what seemed hot oil. I cramped and I knew the nausea would overwhelm me shortly. Each session would end in its own distinct way, but each began with the warm pain, and with the prickling of the fingers. The pain was in the bags, and the bags gave it to me. I began to welcome the urge to vomit, in the hope, always vain, that it would somehow relieve the sickness.

As the terrible episodes continued, my only solace was what I would design in my head. Cold thin air replaced the burning plastic in my nostrils. First I watched the scene high on the glacier from a distance, then I felt what seemed a hundred atmospheres of pressure as I realized it was I climbing on the ice field. I saw crampons grab the snow and move my form forward. Was I near the crest? Sensations of sight and breathing put me on Nisqually glacier, moving to Columbia crest of Mount Rainier. The escape could have been to a relaxed setting, some meadow or lake, but for me to leave the hospital and the treatment behind, the place to go had to be here, this place of challenge. I had to move my struggle elsewhere, to one more familiar, so I went to a place of the final approach to the summit, some 14,410 feet above this hospital room.

The mountain, difficult and dangerous as it is, was still no match for my present reality of chemotherapy. Scents of cold air, fresh in my lungs, gave way to the sensations of acrid chemical odors. Sensations in my head were no longer from the blood circulating in my ears brought on by the rigorous deep breathing of the climb at altitude, but instead by the pounding of the reactions in my blood. I was back in the room.

I could not sleep. Whether it was chemical, psychological, or both did not matter. All that mattered was that I had to find other ways to relax. Entire nights awake followed by cat naps for thirty minutes would carry on for days at a time. It grew worse, and since that time, it has come and gone. Whether the causes were chemical or something else, it was one major challenge that came upon me very rapidly. I felt "sleepless in Tacoma."

In the first week of chemotherapy session, I lost control of my body. The weight seemed to evaporate from my torso, chest, and neck. Muscle mass melted away under the relentless assault of the metabolism induced by the chemicals. I shed thirty-five pounds in one week. Tied to the now hated intravenous pole, the blue box that whirred and whined incessantly, I felt bound by the rope of a tube while it delivered the contents into my veins. The pole cramped me. It got in my way when I went to the bathroom, when I turned in bed. It was both necessary and annoying.

Unlike the people who I met during surgery, the patients I saw in chemotherapy waiting rooms generally did not want to talk very much. People here know they are in for a rough time. Every one in the room has come to some realization about their own mortality. They hope for the doctor to position them in a way to continue to fight the cancer without pain and without damage, but close to the surface is a reflective notion of how they have lived so far. There is also the dose of practical reality that the pain will be theirs alone. They know that very few friends or family can identity with what the chemotherapy is doing to them. They are, in a way, in a divorce process form what they have known so far in their lives. Though I have heard

many people talk about how experience with surgery have turned
out well, I heard little of that with chemotherapy. Maybe that is
because with surgery, there is the underlying idea that something
dangerous and invasive can be removed; while with
chemotherapy that entire premise of it is indirect and mysterious.
While it poisons, the snow keeps you alive, and you wonder if
they really understand it at all. Though the cancer will
camouflage itself to fool you into thinking the tumor is part of
you, the chemotherapy puts on no such illusions. It is there to
hurt you.

Recollections of the feelings have helped me. The recall of
the fear and the pain of each day is a kind of yardstick by which
to understand others in such treatments, by which to remind
myself of how fragile we all are. Back then, I kept wondering
what I was supposed to do with the very vague advice from
doctors, friends, and articles. "It will be a lot easier and go a lot
better it you just relax and it will be a lot better." It sounds
logical, and I always admire those who can use such advice, but
it meant nothing to me until I placed into my own thinking in
ways that might guide some action, and I found that terribly
difficult. I learned later that my instincts which led me to a series
of breathing techniques, followed by meditation, followed by
painting my own pictures in my head, were a part of that action.
But then I did it mainly by instinct. No one described how sick I
should expect to be, and therefore when the sickness began I felt
bewildered. I thought they either betrayed me, which made no
sense, or they truly do not know, which I would find surprising,
or that there was something dangerously wrong with my mixture
of chemotherapy and I was in serious trouble. The last scenario
was what I thought the most likely. And it was mainly because I
simply did not know how ill one person could become.

On the first night in the hospital room, I took no medication,
and did not sleep at all. The chemical treatment bags would be

hung every four hours, and they would begin on my thirty seventh birthday. It was a memorable gift. As the intravenous needle connected to the bag and I saw the drip into the shunt placed in my arm, a wave of heat passed from the hand to the forearm, and up to my shoulder. First it smoldered, then it spread and grew. I was watching the bags, first the chemical bag, then shifting my gaze to the "snow" in the other bag which fed the other arm. I thought I was watching a battle, with me in the center. The heat was not some warm pleasant feeling, not like lying in sunshine, or the feeling of a warm drink on a cold day. Instead, it was a slow, smoldering, dirty fire that put out bilious fumes that sucked into my breathing. Then the image turned to something very distinct, from my recent trip. I thought I was on a tarmac in the Sinai and I was caught behind the jet engine of an aircraft and I could not escape it. The sun burned, the tarmac was like a frying pan, everything burned my eyes, and I could not breathe for the roar of heat blowing into my face. That image built while the physical effects worsened and then I could feel my ears pounding with the race of blood as my circulation goes crazy in the face of the poison. And again I would grow sick to my stomach.

There was no escaping the fear. I tried to think of other things, but the effort to leave was now futile. The nausea would not allow it. I was me trapped in the present reality. Now every drop held a bit of nausea and it all collected in me. As each bag came in every four hours throughout that first day, March 21st, the sickness systematically built. The bags themselves, packed so neatly, labeled so clearly, always balanced so rightly, one bag on each arm, now held my very life in their symmetrical equation around my bed.

I thought I heard a fight announcer. "In this corner, wearing blue trunks, no wait a minute, he isn't wearing any trunks, weighing in at 500 milligrams, from the XYZ Chemical

company in New Jersey, in his 6th bout in the last twenty four
hours, VP 16." The voice continued, "...and in this corner,
weighing another 500 milligrams, from Tacoma Washington,
also in his sixth bout today, "Snow." It was to be a great fight,
and I had to cheer for a draw. I would play the game with myself
for a while. It was the closest I could get to a visualization. Then
I would vomit.

The orderlies and nurses crash into my imaginings. They
look at me, no they are not looking at me, they are instead
looking at the object of their job, the IV pole and the e blue
machine. Someone mention a date last night. Are they talking to
me, to the pole, to themselves? Now they say what they might
have for lunch, where they might go. I wish I could go, but then
get ill when they mention the meal. Then they talk about
something on television and I realize there are two in the room
and she was never talking to me at all. As the recount of
Donahue continues, the needle comes into the arm and the pain
seems sharper. This is not imagination, this is real and it hurts.
The needle into the shunt hurts. Now comes another regime. She
must take another blood test. These are done about four times a
day, maybe more frequently. She sticks the arm and it jams,
pushes, and does not ease into the vein. I tell her she hurts me.
She does not like that fact and tells me that is just "because my
veins are over sensitive "because of the chemotherapy."

I tell her that she is wrong, that it hurts because she wasn't
careful and I tell her I know how an injection for a blood test
should be done, and her angle was too great, and it hurts because
she stabbed me. She does not like this critique, least of all
coming from a patient. "How can he say that?" I hear her say to
someone else. "...how could anyone feel anything with all that in
their veins?" Whether the older lady believes this lie or whether
it is just something they say to each other to pass the day is really
of no concern of mine right now. After the brief bout between us,

she watches the object the bed, me, for the requisite so many minutes (she can get in trouble if they have a bad reaction, another euphemism for being assaulted, then she forces a smile, and turns to the door. I grew angry at the thought that I was an object. Sometimes, I remain angry.

My nostrils fill with a sickening odor that shakes me awake. A foreign, oily substance and out of the corner of my eye I noted a pool of blood on the floor. I hear drips from the pole, but they sound different than usual, and I feel a strange relief. It is blood dripping into a puddle. I start a debate within myself.

Someone will do something; it doesn't need to be me. You won't bleed to death. Don't get up and don't use the call button. If you do, they will come in here and they will make a big thing of it. Then they will blame it on you while you have to stand in the corner, an object, and listen to how you should be more careful with this. They will take forever to make the bed, while you stand with cold feet and cramped stomach and an aching head. And you will have to endure their mutterings....so just lay here.

But another side of me said I must take care of this. I decided to look at the blood again. I reasoned out that I had to clean it up. Setting aside the pain in my gut, I stepped out of bed and avoided the stench in my nostrils, and I took some small pleasure in the fact that the chain of the IV tube was not connected.

Do one thing at a time. Do something. Take charge of something here.

I cleaned the blood from my arm, pulled out the shunt, held a bandage to the wound, and took a deep breath. I then managed myself into the shower and redressed. No help. Finally, when I was satisfied I had cleaned up, I called the nurse. The scene over, I was exhausted, but a good exhaustion, and I slept.

Sleep deprivation held me hostage. It was without a doubt the most difficult part of what I faced in chemotherapy. In the nineteenth century those who ran sanitariums employed devices known as "bird cages" They were iron contraptions that sat on top of the head and shoulders to prevent movement, some attempt to prevent the "patient" from inflicting self destruction. Or so the rationalization of the day argued. I felt like I was in a birdcage. The pain was nearly constant, never allowing me rest. As the weight dropped from my frame, I realized it was not only due to the absence of appetite, but there was some chemical reaction melting the pounds away. By the time the week was done, I had dropped thirty-five of my original one hundred seventy five pounds.

How many times had I been poked, stuck, and tested? The images upon me were not those I would design, but those imposed by the poisons. Any thought of food was overwhelming. Growing weaker each day, my senses changed, and some odors and fragrances that I enjoyed for as long as I could remember were now repulsive. Coffee, cheese, meat, and dozens of other foods normally very appealing were now out of the question.

April 2, 1989 was the day when Debra came to rescue me. Five days of treatment were done, and she came in the room to get me, I had the distinct image of leaving a prison. My return from the Sinai was now a distant memory. This reunion after six days was far more important the one that greeted me after six months. Debra's eyes went wide with shock when she saw me. My weakened and depleted frame suggested all the suffering that I would not speak about. It had only been six days, but how does one measure time? I think my wife dedicated herself to my recovery even before we got into the car. I felt completely helpless and she was there to move me home.

One outcome of chemotherapy is a condition known as nutripenia. It is a name for low white blood cell count, and it is precisely the condition that the oncologist seeks. Doctors cannot precisely measure cancer cell density in the blood, but they can measure the relative count of the white blood cells. The count tells the oncologist how effective was the application of the antineoplastic drugs in the effort to knock down the white count. They reason that if the chemotherapy was strong enough kill those very strong cells, then it probably worked against the cancer cells as well, because the white cells are so involved with the disease. This of course puts the body's defenses at risk, and some common infections such as those caused by the bacteria in fresh food, become very dangerous. An infection will not register a fever, not until the reaction rages so badly that it normally would read 104 or 105 degrees. If any fever is registered at all, I had to go immediately to the emergency room.

The muscles in my neck were cramped for the struggle with the IV pole and the continual tension. The forty pounds that I lost also bared my spine of any fat, and the lack of any cushion prevent any comfort in lying down. No matter how I moved, it hurt. From the pain in my spine and the sores on my skin and the effort to move my neck, sleep and rest became impossible. I walked around the house as if I were doing laps on a track. The next morning, my hair began to fall in clumps. There was the sure sign that all the hair would go: a small clump of hair from a spot the size of a dime came out first. This spot left first and when my hair grew back months later, it was the last to return.

A nurse told Debra about a kind of non-dairy milk. It was developed for hot climates and for long periods of storage with no refrigeration. It is derived from a pasteurization process that captures the nutrients, but not the bacteria. Debra was

determined to find it, but it proved elusive. Even stores that had
heard of it were out of it, and it would be weeks, they said,
before any re-supply. She became obsessed with finding this
supposed new source of my nourishment, and she would
describe for me in detail, at least two or three times a day, how
one store manager seemed to care about this. The commissary
was supposed to carry it, but its demand was relatively rare and
they were simply out of stock for a while. She wrote letters to
companies and to food chains. She drove to Seattle. She did
everything I could imagine to find it, and I did not even drink
milk. I was amazed.

About a year later, while we were walking, she told me with
a light laugh about how she thought each of us dealt with the
cancer.

"Mark, I tried so hard to make you comfortable. I don't
know if you realize how much pain you endured, and this was
one little thing I might do for you. It was like the nights I would
awake at 2:00 AM and cook something because you had a
surprise appetite and taste for a certain food."

"So then it was not about milk at all."

"Only in that the milk was something I could do to feel that I
was not completely helpless. I could do nothing for you, then I
could offer this food, then I could not because no one carried it.
That was what made me crazy."

The nutripenic episodes lasted from March until June. I
would spend about three hours to accomplish these tasks: get out
of bed, walk to the bathroom under my own power, wash my
face, relieve myself, shower, and shave. I would look down into
the sink and had to struggle to lift my head enough to shave. The
neck was not about to handle the weight of my head, and
standing up straight was am major exercise that I forced myself
to do. In the struggle each morning, the nausea would always
return and I had to control it but I had no compass or map to

navigate my way through this course. I had to work my body, but it was not responding, so I worded it anyway. Along with my thinking.

Debra came to me one afternoon and told me that we had to discuss how I would approach the next battle of chemotherapy in the hospital. She told me that I had to do it in a more disciplined way, that I needed a strategy.

"Mark, I want you to write a list of all the things you have to be thankful for, to included the parts of the cancer."

I looked at her like she was crazy. How could she consider the advantages when they still wanted me to continue with chemotherapy? I did not see where this would go and I wanted none of it.

"You got another tumor, true, and the disease spread, true, but they found it and they know where it moved. They really think they got it all. That's point one. Point two is that you have already told the Army you will not put up with a board to dismiss you. You have already made up your mind to get well and to stay in. Point three is that you have us, you have your family, and the kids believe now that you will recover. Make up the rest on your won then let's compare the lists. Do it."

She began to tell me for the first time how all of this was affecting her and how much she wanted to help me. Her instincts told her, even then, that we had to do this together. I had begun to deal with cancer in my own personal ways, but it was time to consider her views as well. I looked past the scars, past the thin layer of skin that now appeared to barely cover bones, and I thought,

What is going on in me? Am I looking at my torso or am I instead looking at some part of my nature, bared to the world? Am I going crazy? Don't. Drink in the picture, now picture a stronger you, one that grows out of what you see.

Now picture the steps along the way to the new you. You will be different.

The effects of surgery and treatments were taking their toll. It would take me some weeks, but I did manage to see myself differently. One vehicle was the preparation for the medical board. When the word came that I required another medical review, I had done my own homework and I told the hospital I would not accept that. I was convinced and my doctors' had told me that there was no reason for me to not recover. Therefore, I now reason to evaluate me for fitness for duty. I argue that I simply had to live within the limits of the profile and recovery on my own and if something happened n my future duty to limit me, then hat would be another matter, to be dealt with later I toured the hospital to support my argument, visiting every doctor who had anything to do with my case. I asked them to evaluate what they wrote about me and they each told me essentially the same thing: that my recovery level would b largely up to me, but it was a relatively unusual request. Most men who have had both testicles removed and all this treatment are fairly anxious to leave the Army. I would then ask if there were some medical reason to expect that I was weakened or that I was at risk for cancer again. The consistent answer was that in medical terms I was free of disease, and then I would politely ask if they could reevaluate their professional judgment and write up a page that said they thought I could retire to duty in time.

I had to regain some control. I was also a reminder of all that the job of the doctors and indeed the purposes of the medical system is to return people to duty, not tot find ways to eliminate them. The first job is to get well. Part of my problem in this was perception. It hovers around the medical language, the terms with which we describe the recovery of patients. When a doctor thinks of a cancer patient being recovered, the system reads that as survival and the absence of disease. There are no provisions within their assumption and their culture of medicine to account for how people feel, or how strong trey may become, or anything beyond the presence or the absence of tumors. They could give me no predictor of the effects of the scarring of the lungs from the chemotherapy, of the amount of energy or fatique I could expect, or of any detail. That would be my business. I asked a series of simple questions as I visited each of them.

"Why do I need a board?'

"What will stop me from recovery?'

"Do you know something you have not told me?"

They each explained to me in their own terms that my body had undergone a various kinds of trauma and that I should be "realistic" about my expectations. None meant to do me or my career harm. But neither did they mean to question any part of the system that surrounds them. In most cases, I have come to find the issue is more about a lack of realization that the patient wants to do more than the prescriptions. Most told me that when they wrote that I should go to a medical board, they did so thinking that is what I would have preferred, to have the leverage to leave the Army if I wanted. They believed, rightly, that the write-ups would influence the advantages of disability payments. That aside, I found that none could say with confidence what we happen next with cancer, what would happen, what side affects. I knew I was in an art as much as I was in a science.

We know how to kill it when we see it, but we don't know where it comes from and we don't know where it goes.

So I decided it would be up to me. Had I tried to leave the Army, or had I asked to leave the infantry, then I would have had the nagging questions of why did I limit myself. My instincts told me to get as well and as fit as I could, even with the risk of working too hard. If I was going to recover as the doctors said nothing medical in my way, then I did not need a board to evaluate whether I should even stay in the army.

As small amounts of strength returned, I found the tips of my fingers and toes became sensitive and painful. My appetite continued to change, but I stuck to the rules of diet: nothing fresh, everything cooked or canned. Food was simply a source of energy for the required work I had to do. I began to exercise. I experimented with stretching routines. Some were very imaginative. I wiggled my body as best I could and I moved as much as I could. The scar down my middle, the length of forty-two staples, meant tightened and painful breathing and moving. I began very disciplined and imaginative stretching routines, taking the appropriate parts of rock climbing conditioning g exercise I had learn, and I practiced disciplined breathing techniques. These were painful, but necessary. My fingers tingled frequently, as if they were constantly asleep. Tingling would turn to pain, pins stabbing at the skin. Finally a welcome numbness would overtake me and I could feel the chemicals moving through my fingers. Cold would follow that, and then I could imagine the glacier.

When the second session of chemotherapy began, I entered the oncology clinic significantly more prepared. I knew what to ask. The mixture I would take this time was and adjustment based on how sick I got the first time. I saw the oncologist more a chemist than a doctor, and I began to understand how it might work. The waiting room of an oncology clinic is a window into a society of the sick and healing processes. My first observation was that the ages in the room ran the spectrum and any notion that cancer was a disease only for the old was dispelled. I thought about most people's reactions to learning of my condition. "But he is so young. He should not get sick." Most simply do not realize that age has little do to with cancer, and unfortunately, most associate cancer with death, and by extension we associate death with aged. But in the waiting room of an oncology clinic those myths are quickly challenged. The oncologist showed me how he was working up a new equation for the "snow." The chemical agents remain in the system for some time after the treatment is over, maybe for life. I began to see the oncologist more as a sorcerer than a doctor, working mixtures with skills of alchemy. His equations mattered much more than my notions about them. But I now saw all of this as fair. It was part of what happened in the world of cancer. The idea that I was only incidental to chemotherapy had invaded my mind and took hold of my spirit. An old friend, Roger Spiller, called me and wanted to know how I was holding up under this onslaught. I was struck that he understood it was an attack, and not just "treatment." I had the privilege of many discussions with Roger, a widely known authority on the psychology and the history of the story of people in war. His work over many years has illuminated a number of facts about the human struggles both great and small that constitute war. He has gift to show emotional and psychological sides of military operations and then show the implications for leadership within all that. He had one memorable statement for me. "You are central to the healing, remember that. Do something with what happened and don't give up."

One might think that my increased knowledge was a great advantage when the next chemotherapy began. But the knowledge also meant that demons, until now bound by my ignorance, were about to be released. My world tightened into sickening odors, pokes in the arm, constraining IV poles. I could not read, could not write, could not do anything but think. I was determined to fight the demons this time. But the experiences from before imparted as much anxiety as they did confidence. I had seen a bit too much of the demons.

I breathed deeply and began to relax. Closing my eyes I fist placed a series of scenes in my head, some from memory some from imagined scenes. The scenes were primarily about me. Each scene was a dream. My friend Marc said to me once that if something is on television, then we think it is important. If the images are never on the screen, then no matter what we think about it at the outset, over time it will not matter to us. If we know that it holds value, then we are frustrated at the interpretation of the value, the image, compare to the real values. So we begin to think, collectively, that our social interpreting and our shared interpretation of what happens to us is so involved with the images captured by cameras.

The images of chemotherapy replay again and again. But my mind, thankfully, did not work like a camera. It took the last interpretation of the trauma and used it. So each time our mind sees an image, we interpret the last image, not the original scene. Television images, no matter how accurate, fool us, because although the scene is real, the context is different from replay to replay. Each time we view a "replayed" scene from the same video, we see it measured not against its occurrence, but measured against our last impression. So we filter and filter our most traumatic images.

The facts of medical recovery are relevant only within the context of the patient's personal and private life. The mind has no power over the medical facts of cancer, but it has enormous power over how those facts are interpreted and used. We can be fooled into thinking that the facts of a case mean that someone will die in six months, then we set our plan to die or to help the patient die, and thereby validate the prediction of the timetable. Or we can reject the notion in part and decide to recover, if the facts are that the disease might allow it. I did not view myself in the mirror as sick and weak, but instead as something against I cold measure progress.

I built newer images of myself. Ones that did not involve
sickness. I used climbing images. On one ascent, my strength
would fail and the rope would leave my hand and I would fall
from the mountain, actually relieved of the need to grip. No
more exhaustion, no more gasping for breath. But then I would
adjust the image and move again into the climb.

Turn it around, turn the pain to the comfort. Like hitting
a baseball, find ways to relax and concentrate.

The ice has a scent and a beauty all its own in its formations
against the pines. It seems to smell like the air itself. The scene is
in my nostrils now and combines with that of the flowers and the
pine of spring at altitude. The odors of cisplatin and burning
plastic were now out of my nostrils and I was back on the
mountain with Elliott. Slowly and heavily, my steps moved
through what felt like water, yet unlike the shaky steps around
the hospital, here on the ice, strangely, they feel secure. With
crampons crunching into the packed snow and ice I noted that
even in the vision my steps were quite short at altitude. The
action is slowed, the effort for so little motion. But motion it
was. The lungs struggle, they burn, the blood does not flow
freely, and for a movement I hold still and breath what I can.
Three breaths later comes another step. My head is aching

Is that the weight of the pack or is the pain of the
position in my bed?

Another three breaths, another step. Talking is out of the
question. So when Elliott, far more fit and practiced at climbing
asks "...Are you all right?' I look down. With Columbia Crest
and the volcanic dome now in sight and moving on the edge of
the ridge, I think nothing of the thousand feet below me. "Are

you all right?" I cannot answer, just walk. Kick the snow, crampon step, flex the knee and lock it past 14,000 feet now and 410 to go. How long, an hour, at least half. No telling. What about that wind? I manage to look up under the weight of the pack and the pain o altitude and five the answer, but when I do it is not the climbing partner. A nurse asks, "...are you all right?" I am back.

The tips of all ten fingers are numb. Arms have no feeling hands are again all done. Look for them, find your hands. Try to feel them. Muscles are cramping again. I struggle to keep eyes closed, but it is no use. Must give up the pain of the climb for the pain of the bed. I return to the bed and the chemicals, but only for r a time.

Though difficult and dangerous, the mountain's course in my mind was no match for challenges beside my bed. Gone was the healthy strain of the weight of the mountain pack. In its place was the familiar pain camouflaged, the pain that deceives as it builds in neck and shoulders. It tells you it will not go, and it will lead to nothing good. This is pain for the sake of itself. I must yield to its power, and I cry out. I move between the two; the pain of the mountain and the pain of the bed.

I returned to scenes of rock and snow again and again. With each visit to the scene, I added some detail, so that the picture formed over time to a healthy image. The scenery was always amidst height. The message is always about clear and cold atmosphere. When I enter the picture, I am calm and feel confident and strong, but the fingers always tingle. My hospital bed, no matter my scenery, will not be denied completely.

On the last night in the hospital, I walked again, and felt the connections to the mountain in even greater detail and strength. Awake all night again, but gone were the aches. Somewhere, I slept.

On a day shortly after being home, I wanted real air, and I went outside to walk. I had not been out on my own in months, and something told me to go. A rain surrounded me, but I walked. Then the scar reminded me this was not a vision, but a wound, and I needed to turn back. I was three miles away from home, and the panic began to overtake me. But I breathed and put myself somewhere on the mountain again. And it worked. The panic came and left.

My fingers and toes were still numb and no hair had returned. My muscle density and strength were still absent, and everything was very unfamiliar from what I felt before. It was like playing with a new body, a new set of lungs, muscles, and limbs.

Nutripenic conditions were passing and that I was recovering, I felt like I could beat all this again. In spite of the numbness and the minor physical limitations and ailments, I was going to get better all the way. It was time to understand the cancer. It was also time to leave this place.

Did I beat this? If so, then how?

I went to the rocks. The day spoke of spring. Once while out on a peak, when I could not figure the way to go and felt frozen, my friend reminded me that climbing was simply movement. Now on this May afternoon in the wake of what happened, I did not care about past and future. I wanted only this time and place. The "art of vertical ballet" appealed to me. I did not climb in the best of form, and I tired sooner than I would have liked to admit, but I did as the surgeons instructed. I began to move.

6 WEST AND EAST

Wes' eyes, bright enough to dance for brief moments, were the only parts of him that I recognized. A year earlier he was the picture of health, all six feet four of him strong and vibrant. But the cancer that began in his colon moved rapidly, and he could no longer claim his health as his just reward of his personal war. Now, the only visible sign of his temporary victory over his own cancer was the sack that was surgically affixed to his side.

As we pulled the car into his driveway, a lady drove up behind us. She told us she was a home nurse, and came to place a shunt into Debra's father's side. "The pain gets worse every day," she said with a little more exasperation than kindness. "This will let us put the pain killers and the chemotherapy to work faster. The doctor will probably give him cannabis next week. That will help."

"Cannabis," I repeated silently. "Efforts to level out the pain with the marijuana derivative. Nothing to offer to cure or to prolong life, only something to relieve pain. *We will poison you, but we won't hurt you...*" When the doctors begin to ease the pain, they are processing him through to death. I made no judgment on that. That may be all they can do. But even before I left the car, I knew he was dying.

We traveled to Utah hoping to celebrate with Wes and Lisa, Debra's parents. Life had suddenly begun anew for us, with my clear recovery and the ides that I had beaten this, but it was just as suddenly changed back into a new set of traumas. For Debra, visions of me facing cancer were only weeks old when her father presented the picture of a man at his end. Even before we entered the house, we both sensed that the elation over my recovery had ended, here in this driveway.

"He needs the shunt so the morphine can get to him quicker, but I don't think it will do much good much longer," the nurse continued. "The pain is gaining on him every day."

I had grown to know him through the years of my marriage to his oldest daughter, and I knew that the attention had shifted away from me before we even got into the house. My honeymoon with the emotional highs of recovery had just ended and in that moment, selfishly, I hated this place, this time.

Since his cholostopy and chemotherapy treatments many had held hope that that the effects of the colon cancer would soon pass, so when they learned about my chemotherapy, no one told us about Wes. That is the way with cancer; it is faithful only to its own fickle character.

I helped my mother-in-law take him to the doctor, and my private world of health and happiness was shattered. The doctor told us that the cannabis he prescribed was strictly for the pain, and that it was only a matter of time before the liver or the spleen was involved, and then he would die. I noticed that visitors talked about him rather than to him, a sign that people expect death. They seem to say, "Do you know when it will be? How soon? We hope you don't put us through too much trouble. We know you are dying, but you see, well, we have so much else going on and if you could just get this over with, we would really appreciate it." Most people do not accept the dying, and therefore tend to put the condition into terms of the living that tell us that life is forever precious. Most people simply do not know how to act, what to do, when confronted with the realty that we die. The result can be cruel. The patient's bed is a gathering place for others to socialize, and dispense their own remedies for the troubles of life, while the one who is sick grows more marginal with each passing day.

His pain was incessant, but he had lucid, clear thoughts. Humor would pop out now and then. I looked beyond the temporarily withering body, beyond the skin that now struggled to hold back the ever-advancing tumors. I was not afraid of the image in front of me, and I was not holding on to a time now gone. I chose to see him in another time, when his strong frame and his skilled hands saved a day for me. We were in the hills above his beloved Cache Valley, where he would delight in the picture and the scent of paintbrush flowers in a mountain meadow. Both pictures of him, the one in the bed and the one in the mountains were valid. I chose to see the one in the mountains. I thought of how he taught me to communicate without speech and my mind muted the room's chatter.

The scents of sage and milkweed were among us in the late afternoon. Dust was golden in the sunlight. It had been one of those remarkable days when I felt as connected to this land as I did to the streets of the Bronx. Sean was seven years old. My many trips here produced a welcome familiarity. But it was Wes that held me here. He was a remarkable man. We shared interests in everything, it seemed. We had gathered the three Arabian horses at his mother's house, a vestige of an era now passing from this part of the country, its beautiful contrasts of high desert and mountains painted on the horizon. Utah began as home to settlers, Mormons who saw the valleys visions of prophets, and this young religion built a great respect for the land into the people. The signs of this belief are all over the west, and one such is in the irrigation of the farms along the valley floors. Wes maintained what was left of his mother's farm with his share of a water system ingenious for its simplicity, and he worked his garden on this mini-ranch every evening. He would take me there on each visit, and together we would care for the place with the chores.

We loaded the horses into the trailer, drove into the hills. The day settled into a series of ridge walks, canters, and an occasional light gallop and we rode for hours. Sean settled into the familiar comfort of the crux of his grandfather's secure hold around the saddle. Ease and confidence were written all over the trio; Wes, Sean, and Bess the horse. Some distant memory planted in my muscles many years tried vainly to get me to handle my horse with the same ease, but I recalled that I always had to work at this, while it seemed that Wes and Sean shared the genes for it.

We rode until the sun was low against the ridges of the Wasatch Range, then made our way back to the trailer. In the time it took to dismount the three horses and collect them into the trailer, the magic was about to change to terror.

I sensed the snake before I heard it. The nervousness in my horse is probably what told me. My eyes searched for the trouble, hoping that it was far away, an avoidable obstacle. But the scene was badly arranged for that. The pickup truck, just connected to the trailer, separated the two Arabians, with Sean in between them, from Wes and me. I still had the rope on the paint, and I led him to a tree some ten feet on our side where I tied him quickly when I saw the some of the six-foot timber rattler. Our eyes agreed on the first move.

Think, don't talk. Cue on Wes. Take your signals from him, from his eyes. Watch him and do what his eyes tell you. He is not talking, so you don't talk. Don't call out to Sean, not yet. He has the better view, the better angle. He will lead here.

One snake was coiled, and from the noises we knew there was at least one more under the brush. Had we somehow stumbled into a nest? We seemed to be somewhere in the center of them. Three very nervous horses, one of which held Sean, and two equally nervous humans.

Get something here under control. Follow his eyes.

By all rational expectations, at least one of us, probable Sean, should have been either bitten and maybe died by one of the snakes, trampled by one of the three very large, strong, and very panicky horses, or driven off the side of the cliff forced by a horse. Instead, a synchronized series of movements took place. The horse trailer was hitched to the pickup. I was on one side, Wes on the other, and the horse that Sean sat atop was directly behind the trailer.

He has the better view, he has the lead. Follow him.

His eyes told me to move first to Sean, even if it meant stepping across the rattler. It was risky, but it was the only clear shot. Any attempt at going for the snake first would surely spook the amazingly strong and fast animal, and she take off with Sean, certain to throw him. So, while we still had some time, someone had to get Sean down and then move the horses out of sight of the rattlers. By our relative positions that task fell to me. Somewhere in my mind I asked how I got into this crazy situation, but then let the thought go.

Like a boxing match. Figure the combinations, set it in your head, rehearse it like dance steps in the head, then do it. See each move. Miss nothing. When you move, do not hesitate. See all the moves, then do them in your head, then do them. Your left foot will take a long step, then your right foot will move off toward the far right, on to that rock, then you will pivot and jump at once and reach up and grab him. Use both hands, and even if you are bitten, you must continue once you have him. Move him from the horse hold him high up, and put him inside the bed of the truck. Then return to the horse and grab her bit and calm here. You can do it.

My own father's story... A man gets a different view from a horse, Mark, a better view.

We each knew what to do without speaking. That is what I always missed about him. Whenever away form him, that trusted confidence that you always knew what to do when around him, without talk. At least I did. I moved slowly and as much as possible at an angel to the snake and as it moved one way I crossed its path from the rear and I made it. It turned and hissed, but I had already taken Sean down and launched him, half throwing him, into the bed of the pickup, the safest place, scary, because it meant moving him toward the diamond back rattle snake, but to safety nonetheless. That done, I guided the sleek Arabian back thirty feet and tied her to a tree in a new direction.

Wes herded the other two horses, and when we both agreed that horses and Sean was safe, we went after the snakes. Instincts told me to let them go, but with three snakes in our midst, instincts alone would not work. Herding snakes is not something to practice, and neither of us was sure how to do it, but with our eyes locked and we agreed to move in the same direction.

When it was over, we did not speak of it. We knew that we
were both "good and lucky" as a team that evening.

Back in the present, again at his bedside.

Someone in the living room was talking about how they
thought the president was going to kick Noriega and all
communists out of Nicaragua. They said the "liberal press"
should just leave the heroes who sell arms to the contras alone.
The talker wanted to know what I as a "military man" thought
about all that. I got up and left the house, feeling absolutely
alone. I only wanted to see my father-in-law in some kind of a
miraculous cure.

Later that evening, when the visiting nurse brought the
"medicine" for the shunt, I grew nauseous. Again, I was
transplanted in time, not to a mountain trail, but this time to the
hospital. It was two weeks earlier, and I was there for my final
treatment for bleomycin. My mind turned back the clock the
weeks that now seemed decades to the picture of another set of
tubes, another shunt, these going into my veins.

*Transposed again in time and space, I was three weeks
in the past, in the oncology clinic where the poison enters me
so that I may heal. Will it heal me or must I heal myself?*

I sat under the nurse's watchful eye while she injected the
bleomycin into the shunt in the top of my wrist. The treatment
continued once a week for several weeks after my release from
the in-patient phase of chemotherapy. I was to sit and wait while
the intravenous needle was inserted with the chemical. So much
sitting. So much waiting. Just as before, it was mainly the
product of chemical calculations designed to produce the final
effects on the carcinoma. But I had enough of seemingly endless

"simple procedures," that I lost control of myself. It was one of those days when it all seemed too much. This last session intersected with our move to West Point, New York, and I somehow began to attach unrealistic significance to it. Philosophically, the treatments represented the last steps that would allow me to leave all of this behind. A comforting, if unrealistic notion.

Don't use the disease as a crutch, don't let it win. But also don't wish it away. Instead, use it. Go back to him, back to the present.

I had recently absorbed chemotherapy, uncertainty about any future in the Army, chemical imbalances from the beginnings of testosterone replacement. But nothing compared to his death.

Back on the oncology ward, back in Washington, the nurse is starting the drip drip into the hand again. The pinprick seems to hurt more than before. Why does it always hurt? When will the hurting stop? I cannot watch when they stick me any more. But I must just sit and wait.

My knowledge of the effects of the drugs might lead the uninitiated to think that since I knew something of chemotherapy, it might be easier to take. But the effect was quite the opposite. My memory, vivid and clear, caused me to balk even at the sensation of the sticking of the needle. The sickeningly warm fluid moving up the hand, up the arm, then into the mouth. A faint distinct taste in the mouth, a little shortness of breath. My emotions went wild with me again and I lost control. I was tired of coming to the doctor for these kinds of things. I was tired of the pokes and sticks, of being treated as an object. I wanted to be out in the sunlight, to walk away from here.

"Why are you hurting me?" I asked the nurse.

"I'm not hurting you. This should not hurt."

"Don't tell me what should not hurt. It does. How much longer do I need to stay here? I want to leave."

"That isn't up to me. I need to take you to the oncologist when we are done."

The last bleomycin treatment produced a new label for me, "free of disease." The term is not "cured" because the standard for cure of cancer is quite high, usually expressed in a number of years without incident of recurrence. Debra shared in the elation for a short time, but soon after the news came the visit to her father. His colon cancer stopped us cold. She was in a sea of contrasts. She was denied the knowledge of her father's deteriorating medical condition, yet everybody was aware of the very private condition of her husband.

On the oncology ward again. I begin to panic. Sweat pouring off of my brow, I felt my heart quicken in pace, and I almost could not believe my ears. I would not go to see the doctor again, I told myself. No need to go back into that waiting area. I can't take it now. Any other time, but not now. Now I need to breathe. The waiting area is not for me, I am better now. I don't want to go there any more. And I won't.

It was over now; the last treatment of bleomycin is done. You will have no more chemotherapy. At least not for now.

Back to the bed, and back to Debra, now having moved from her husband's sick bed to her father's.

It was as if her validity as a person, her very ability to take charge of her own life was challenged. The challenger was not some societal prejudice or vague notion of misapplied justice, but the whims of cancer cells that invaded her life on at least three fronts: her husband, her plans for children, and now her father. Nowhere was the wreckage of the whims of cancer cells felt so strongly. She was close to her limits on several fronts, and my ability to help was rapidly drained by the same scenarios. That was Debra, always pushed to her limits, always coming through.

Another part of Debra's outlook began to come to the surface. The assumption then was that the one testicle was not a threat to my virility and that the spread to other testes was highly unlikely. Therefore, the "guardian ball" that I wrote about earlier in radiation treatment was considered sufficient to save the sperm production of the other testicle. But it never occurred to me or my wife to visit a sperm bank in the event that something went wrong. Debra now had the added pressures of a lack of sympathy or understanding as to why she was sad over the loss of children that might have been. Most who knew read the attitude as a bit selfish, whereas in reality it was simply another feeling of loss. Everyone sees the invasion of cancer through their own lenses, and each of us had to heal in our own ways.

Not far from where the scene with the horses played out three years earlier, Sean and I found our way to a spot above the town where we looked out over Cache Valley. The irrigation ditch held water that cooled us a bit on this very hot and very still afternoon. He was eleven years old. He knew that our trip was no longer about a visit to his grandpa's house, was no longer about a move to West Point. It was no longer about a vacation to celebrate his Dad's return from the hospital. Now the visit was about dying. I took him on a long hike to a place in the valley that he remembered quite well. I took them camping and fishing.

One afternoon on one of our walks, I was talking about something along the way when Sean looked at me and said,

"Is Grandpa going to die?" he asked.

"Yes."

"Why is he going to die? You told me that people don't have to die from cancer, that they can get better. You did."

"There are different kinds of cancer, Sean, and sometimes the only thing about them that is the same is simply the word cancer. The kind of cancer your grandpa has is very different and very much more dangerous than mine. I was lucky that the kind they found in me could be treated. His is different."

Explaining this to my eleven-year-old son was no more or less difficulty than explaining it to adults. People die from cancer when cells grow into tumors and when tumors invest a vital organ. The body does not read the tumor as an invader, and when the therapy goes to work the body's immune system takes over and rejects the vestiges of the cancerous cells, but only after chemotherapy or radiation has begun the job. When it all works right, the body itself devours the cancer. When it does not work, though, the cancer takes over and transforms the healthy into he sick once again.

One evening, while he struggled to sip some liquid, he began to talk about going. He wanted me to take some of his fishing and hunting things, he said. He began to give things away. It became a little easier for everyone then, everyone except Sean.

We left Utah and went to Debra's sister's home in Wichita. After waiting a week with no word, we continued on to New York. A tornado greeted us on the George Washington Bridge and we turned onto the Hutchinson River Parkway to the Saw Mill River Parkway to re unite with my childhood friend and his family, Marc Guthartz in White Plains. But the tornado was nothing to what awaited us at Marc's house. Deb's mother had left a message to call; Wes died that morning.

I had a feeling on that one summer day in White Plains that I was not only recovering, but actually physically stronger than ever before. My friend Marc and I jogged one day and my strength seemed to come very easily. I knew that I was merely feeling good for the day, that it would be some time before I could really expect the full return of my strength, it at all. But I thought that it was back. We ran for about forty minutes, and I felt very strong. I felt strong, and that was all that mattered to me. I asked my friend a question that surprised both of us.

"Marc, Do you think you could start your life over?"

"What do you mean, start over?"

"I mean that I think I have changed."

"Well, you look a little heavier, but you don't mean physically do you?"

"No, I don't. I mean that I have to change something in me, something I can't define right now, but something I sense. I mean that I think I got cancer a second time because I did not understand it when I got it the first time."

"So what do you want to do now?"

"I don't know, exactly, but I think I need to do something with the cancer. It feels like it's right to begin again, to start over without the baggage of the past. What would you do if you could just sell your business and start over somewhere and something else? Would you?"

"What baggage?" he asked me cautiously, a cautious tone that says "be careful how you answer this, it may be a test question that counts."

I had no answer. The baggage was the disease. He was my oldest and closest of friends and he was careful to both listen and guide, to allow me to discover for myself what was at work here. The idea of starting something over, of recapturing something lost, was strong in me. It was much more significant than, it was somewhere in the self ideas and the luggage I carried within me

that though they accompanied me for many years to all points on
the map, they remained were nevertheless unexamined.

"So what about you, Mark, what if you could do anything
with yourself right now. What is it?

I rolled the thought around in my mind before I said, 'I think
I would do exactly what I'm doing."

The clarity of thought arrived like a dancer in a chorus line
who emerged into the spotlight for a moment and crystallized the
story, then returned just as quickly to the camouflaged
anonymity of the crowd. But the thought was worth the wait to
see the solo dancer. I sensed that I would find the clarity, or that
it would find me, again soon. The ideas that play hide and seek
always seem to dance around us.

"So, you want to do exactly what you are doing?"

"For now. Yes. But I will say that I now see things in time
very differently now. I see one time leading into another."

We took our five boys to Yankee Stadium. Down the Bronx
River Parkway on the Cross Bronx Expressway, we passed Third
Avenue, Southern Boulevard, and Webster Avenue.
Neighborhoods. When we got to the Stadium, I recalled the *Field
of Dreams* story, the idea that you can go back and capture a
time to correct some wrong. But my feelings were not solely
philosophical. They were also practical. I would leave the game
early to receive Debra at Laguardia Airport after her return from
her father's funeral. I should have been there with her, I thought.

The five of us were in the upper deck on the third base side.
An old favorite spot from which you can look down and out.
Scents, old familiar scents wafted up from the field and in from
the water. The hot dogs, beer, and that special smell of big
league grass in a place surrounded by city air with a cool
summer evening breeze off the Harlem River mixed in
remarkable. No odor made me ill. I took in the game, absorbed
it, drank in the motions, the artful ballet-like precision with

which a pro ball player simply throws. I saw things I never saw
before in Yankee Stadium. I saw dance and geometry, and real
beauty. I watched the game and seemed to see much more than
the game on the field, somehow I saw the future in my mind.
Baseball is not about what is happening, but rather about what
might happen next; a game of pregnant moments. It is the art of
the possible, representing some future action much more than
depicting what is happening in the present. But it was time to get
Debra, and I left early.

I had parked the car on 159th Street to recover my car and
my internal compass guided me left onto the Grand Concourse,
connecting streets to Mosholu Parkway, passing fields where I
played baseball. On a spontaneous notion, I drove through our
neighborhood, past my mother's house, and took the streets up to
the connecting roads to the airport. Bronx Park East into Burke
Avenue, up passed the familiar street names; Throop,
Bronxwood, Colden, across the Boston Post Road, a right turn
on to Gun Hill Road and then the connection again to a spur of
Interstate 95 to the Bronx Whitestone Bridge into Queens. I kept
the window open to get a sense of the sound, the smells, and the
words that are the city. A sense of familiarity, if not complete
community, enveloped me as I navigated. It was like an old
friend knocking on my door.

Flipping the radio stations from "News Radio 88, WCBS" to
some "jazz only" station, WQEW, where I found Frank Sinatra. I
recalled once again the substance that was here. The announcer
was explaining some recording session in 1965 when Sinatra and
Nelson Riddle mixed the song "Days of Wine and Roses." "Only
here," I said to myself, can you hear this."

The Whitestone Bridge is among the most handsome spans I
have seen anywhere. Its relatively tall towers seem always to
gleam and its high arc stands in contrast to its sister Throggs
Neck Bridge and the older uglier brother the Triboro. As I

crested its center and picked up the road sign for "Route 678 and New York Airports," The bridges we would need had to span gaps that had little do with rivers or geography. When I saw her face, I knew she had been to her own hell. While I had been spending the weeks engaged in some vague and idealistic notions of my future, Debra was right now tied inextricably to the past. I wanted to be there with here, could not, not now. How strange, I thought, that in a matter of seconds, I have sensed that there would be a gap between us for months and I did not know how to bridge it, not now. While she would need to mourn death while I wanted to celebrate life.

Once again, the contrasts struck me. I never felt so deeply in love, yet so distant. It seemed to me that we needed a kind of semi permanent divider between us; a filter, something that would allow each of us to privately guard our feelings while also enabling us to connect.

"Mark, all I can say is that his pain is now gone. But I already miss him. He should not have died."

Again, no answers, only the willingness to ask questions, to not give up.

Where is the cancer? In cells or in my mind? Why does it matter at all? Matters in relation to the references I set in my head. Might matter to others.

It was easy to get started at West Point. My work and fun were completely connected. It was a kind of playground, and I chose to see positive aspects of it. So much to me seemed connected to things permanent, in clear contrast to the nomadic nature of most of Army life. So much here was connected to rock and to height. With my second surgery and the removal of the remaining testicle, came a new challenge of hormone replacement. Testosterone is an anabolic steroid that aids in sexual functions and maintains male characteristics. Body hair, tone of voice, and muscular density among the most obvious. I began to take injections of an enthalate form of it, a derivative of animal chemicals. In the months after surgery, this became a major adjustment and I decided to make informal measurements of my athletic activity, my relative level of fatique or endurance, and my muscle mass and strength. Normally, the brain sends signals based on the expected activity to the testes that tell them how much to produce. Such messages are balanced against the natural levels of estrogen and the steroid is released into the systems to instigate growth or sexual activity. In my case, I had to learn how to space the injections to regain some sort of balance over the two or three week period over which the injection substituted for my natural testosterone production.

I had designed exercise regimes to build muscle and flexibility and regain the lost lung capacity that I experienced after the chemotherapy. After some months of disciplined and regular work, it began to fit together: the balance of aerobic, anaerobic exercises and the shots. I studied something of exercise physiology and about performance training, and I used a great deal of variety as I tried to build strength and maintain regular weight.

It was based on the use of approximately one hundred milligrams per week, taken in either three or two week intervals. Because I had grown so shy of needles and pain, I began the replacement therapy with the three-week variety. I found that my shoulders, chest and arms increased in size and I was gaining weight, and my emotions were running very high. I elected to go on two-week cycles which leveled out the effects. The shots caused me to develop a tendency to gain weight, most of which was muscle mass. My new interest in climbing caused me to seek out flexibility training, and in that way climbing became a way for me to go where I could not go before.

The rock climbs for me would connect mind and body, and give me the notion that I could play with gravity. It was a vehicle to allow me to get well. One day on a wall, my fingers became completely numb. Panic set in first, then confidence as I found a way to move my hands despite no senses. As I negotiated the moves within the pitch, my partner, a cadet, could not see that I was in trouble. I told myself I had no safety rope and thought my way through the e relatively easy, but nonetheless technical route. I was numb, on a ledge, and in the safety of my own ability.

Like most of what happened in this story, our time at West Point was filled with contrasts. In the summer of 1990, the training program that I was part of designing and running was the center of my life. It represented everything right and good with the Army. We had put a lot of planning into the program to connect it to the soldiers in the Army and we got them up to West Point, and they do every year. I needed this project to go for more reasons than the job or the responsibility for training the cadets. I needed it because it was the first thing of substance that I did since the cancer.

The announcement of my selection for battalion command, a milestone in the career of any officer, took on even greater moment for me since the recovery. It was a validation, official recognition by the system of the Army that what I knew for myself, that I was well. Even in the face of the physical profile that was now a part of my record, the board selected me for battalion command I expected to remain at West Point through the following summer, but scenarios of troop movements to the desert meant that many things were changing rapidly, and that had to change to a short notice move. And in the fall, when its beauty is unmatched, and when I had just begun to reacquaint with friends and family all over that area. I did not want to leave West Point. It became the place of my recovery, my re-entry into the human race. It was the place where I healed. Awaiting the word about where to go next is never easy in the Army, but this move was especially hard. This was the place of my recovery. I did not want to move. With the summer and the training also came Desert Shield begun, I waited. Then I learned we would go to Fort Benning, Georgia, in October of 1990.

Balanced against the physical beauty of the Hudson Valley and of West Point itself was another tug at my heart. We arrived one year earlier, in the summer of 1989, twenty years almost to the day that I entered the Academy as a plebe. Now, I would depart again, finally having learned and applied something that might have been a great tragedy, my cancer, into a place of value in my life. That realization was illuminated in this very special and magical year at West Point, and it related to what I learned there as a cadet. I had learned how to play myself. I had learned to rock climb, and climbing as they say, is moving in a whole new direction. It would be very hard to leave here so suddenly. West Point attracts and holds, and it is not an easy place to leave. It formed a very warm and welcome protective shell around our family for the past year. We had expected to go in the following summer, but the Army's burdens of change as it met the needs of the forces in the Saudi desert meant that many schedules changed and changed rapidly. The word came for me to go sooner, just a month or so after the summer training ended.

October and West Point always seem wedded. It is never easy for me to leave there, but it especially difficult at the height of fall. There was a chilled freshness in the air and every smell, sight, and sense of West Point begged me to not leave. The reds, golds, and were alive and brilliant in the light from the sun's low angle. The place tried to hold me again, but we drove away, to the South.

7 "PAINT MY HOUSE"

How does one prepare for the onslaughts? The personal moral codes, methods of thinking, emotions and spirit that help people to gather the strength are all a part of what a recovering patient uses. But I have found that other tools, designed for particular purposes, worked far more effectively than general and moral guidelines. At first without any intended purpose, then later with what seemed born more out of instinct than any learned skill, I crafted such implements to fill the gaps between the cancer and myself. To live and recover, I had only to follow the doctors' instructions. But to heal, to get well, I found that I needed to explore the connections within myself as well as the links within the cancer.

From a practical perspective, one of the first things to do is to get the person to a comprehensive cancer treatment facility. They are available nearly everywhere in the United States. Rather than rely solely on the advice of the entry point to health care, the patient should investigate all aspects of medical treatment for their kind of cancer. Help a friend by finding the resources.

I found that commonly used analogies such as "battle," and "war" were of little use. Once the cancer and the treatments visited upon me effects I did not expect; overwhelming sickness, weakness, questions of my future and the effects on my family, well worn code words meant little. Perhaps doctors find utility in the phrases for they design weapons, strategies, and tactics to destroy enemies on whom they have gathered important intelligence, and they treat the cancer as an invasive enemy. But the comparisons were too narrowly focused for me, and they left large parts of me untouched. The mix of desperation and elation that I felt could not be explained by anything short of a careful, deep look in the mirror.

In my first case of cancer, I saw the struggle in direct ways, as if I was in a boxing match; my pugilistic skills applied in my characteristic straightforward style against my opponents' powerfully indirect methods. I had studied nothing of the theory and learned little about the practice of experiences with cancer. As the treatments progressed, my methods, born only of instinct, proved vague and only loosely developed. If there was a definable enemy, it was not in the cancer cells alone, but also in my own psyche. Cancer is cells gone crazy, and because the body's own healthy cells have been transformed into cancerous ones, the body must transform once again, not "back to what it was," but into something very different from what it was before the cancer.

Interactions within the body cause the cancer to spread, and to consider it a contest of "winners" and "losers," would then have clearly been too narrow a view. It would not have accounted for Wes, a man who was in every respect the example of the hardest and craftiest of fighters and one that had a remarkable capacity for love. The strongest of people, he could do nothing to hold back the disease's claim on him as it grew like a weed in his system. But it took me years to study and understand, and then accept this; the idea this was not about winners or losers, but rather about what we do with disease when it happens. Maybe one can recapture a time past, at least in the use of it for the future. If I could have recaptured a time and done something with it. What would that be?

This is a brief description of how I would have liked others to see me as I went through what I did. I found strong messages about disease all around me. Most of the signals drive people away from facing illness. It engines vague notions of "getting back to your old self." When I recovered from my first case, I worked hard to do what most people expected; I followed the conventional wisdom and went back to what I was before. The expressions illuminate the ideas that we should avoid and reject the illness. We tell ourselves to put it away, to forget it. It is done, never to be used again, probably never even discussed again. Much of the messages concern how I looked. "You look good as new," "He looks like his old self," "He doesn't look sick." The messages seek to protect the well from the knowledge of the sick by creating the image that everyone is trying to become as healthy as they were before. In fact, one could argue that the clinics are filled with people who are to be treated to gather medical information or to serve the wealthy who support the hospitals as long as the research continues.

In each of my cases, early detection was a major factor in the outcome. In my first case, the growth on the testicle began a few months before my routine visit to the doctor, and I never realized it might be a tumor at all. I thought that if it was anything, it was an infection. The warning signs of testicular cancer are clear: any growth, pimple, or knot on the testicle, usually on the surface. Sometimes it is accompanied by other symptoms such as swelling and pain, but not always. In my case, the knot was there for several months, and I simply did nothing about it, out of my own ignorance of the disease. Therefore, the growth was allowed to go on for some time. Luckily, it remained contained. Had it been another, more aggressive cell, having it go untreated for so long probably would have contributed to it spreading.

With no small amount of irony, two years later the second tumor was detected at a very early stage of its development. Once again, it was a doctor who detected it, and not me, but this time it was not for lack of trying. I was doing self-examinations. It was simply that I was scheduled for follow up examinations. The blood tests for tumor makers caused no alarm. The growth had not yet secreted into the blood to the level that would indicate any abnormal levels. It was only the experienced urologist who detected that a tumor had again begun to grow.

Tactics and strategies do not always clearly align. So it is in cancer. The first question was one of objective, what is it that we were to shoot for. Was it *"total cell eradication?"* Or was the objective something short of that? If it was, then the next question might reasonably be, "Is this a new tumor or is it some vestige, something undetected before?" If was the second case, then the problem would appear to be significant, because testes tumors of seminoma do not spread from side to side. Instead, they spread up into the system of lymph nodes and possibly into the area of the chest. If it did not spread from the other side, then it is some kind of a completely new case. The strategy was to get it all, every last remnant of every growth and every cell of what might be left after they all my nodes were removed.

The surgeons see the final goals, if not always the tactics along the pathways. They attack the tumor, whatever its stage, with weapons as potent as the patient can sustain to achieve total cell kill. In my case, they concluded that nature of the tumor was clearly aggressive, and it demanded aggressive treatment. Through the lenses of medicine, it was very logical. But for me, there was great fear and visceral reactions, despite all the logic. My questions were about how long would all this take, how much more pain and limitations will be involved, what about my upcoming move. How long will I be in the hospital? At every turn, there was a new question of what would come next.

Is cancer in our genes or is it in our mind? As uncertain as where it begins, it is equally certain that it resides and grows in our cells. As the days passed, my emotional feelings were heightened, and my first challenge was the enormous, almost overwhelming sense of being alone. It was a thought that I found at once fascinating and frightening, and it tore at my emotions.

Cancer is "cells gone crazy," and cells are hard to visualize as powerful forces in one's life. They are too small for us to know well, and cancer's greatest paradox may lie in that its scale and size holds such enormously threatening power. My body's mysteries washed over me, and I did not realize the intricate details of the blood and lymphatic systems. They are simple in their complexities. So intricate is the body that at points in the system, capillaries become so narrow that blood cells actually move through them in single file. As small as it is at its extensions, the system has a relative vastness. It would stretch out for miles if unfolded from its storage position within the body. And as many times as the lymphatic and blood systems fill and refill, its efficiencies remain nearly miraculous. The blood accounts for only ten per cent of the body's volume, but it covers virtually one hundred per cent of its area.

Some five years after the treatments, an illustration of the complexities came to me in the form of a real scare. I found a distinct lump in my neck, in the area of a lymph node. The doctors did extensive tests, including g another CT scan, and tumor markers, and the node was definitely a little more than just swollen. A urologist who had just recently studied some effects of belomycin told me about recent findings that chemotherapy patients who have been treated with bleomycin experience similar scares, and the theory is that if one microscopic point in the blood were selected, and followed through the entire system, then in about five years it would return to the same spot in the system. When a small part of bleomycin moves through the system, it may settle, for a time, in a node and it creates the appearance of a problem. But the chemicals do not leave the body and they pass the same point in the circulatory system every so many years.

From transformed cells, the disease can move anywhere in the body's lymphatic or circulatory systems to settle, for a time in a place where it may be exposed long enough to be attacked. Depending on the nature of the cell and the location of the tumor, the general area to where it might spread can be predictable.

But do we ever kill it? Do we ever eradicate the cells? We do not. For the cells are a part of us. And once again the patient, as well as the doctors are faced with the art, even the philosophical, as much as they are the science. The fight is not against some definable invader whose outline is clear and the fight is not static. The body itself is, chemically and clinically as well as spiritually, a series of flowing movements, a series of rivers, and the cancer is something in the flow, somewhere in the flow of the stream.

I found that my personal code of behavior did not stand up to the treatments. Notions of what to do and of how to act were a bit too rigid for the very nimble and quick moves that the disease visited upon me. I was mistaken in my outlook on my own body, and my health. I focused on motion and activity and performance; and not very much on nutrition, rest, and the biofeedback and mental aspects of conditioning or preparation. I had not put any personal stamp on the connections between body and mind, and especially between body and spirit. Training in various sports and in the intense parts of the Army provided little more than a certain level of self-confidence. But toughness means little within the context of chemotherapy treatment. As the chemicals flow, so do the body's systems, and I began to reason that my spirit as well as my mind must also find a way to move in conjunction with this flow. If I remained static in any aspect of my body or sprit, then it seemed me that I would again be vulnerable.

I used techniques of visualization, physical training, meditation, and prayer. My initial feelings and reactions to the physical pain were valid, but they were not sufficient to sustain me. I focused on the pain, then taught myself to meditate in order to overcome it. I would take real scenarios and overlay on them on scenes I imagined, mixing the best of what I experienced with the best of what I could imagine. In a moment, I was out of the bed, and on a trail, a park, a city street and cafe. The scenery kept moving it seemed and every change in my condition seemed to instigate a change in backdrop and I leaned to keep a little bit ahead of the pain. Although my focus on pain led me to think that this was all about me and although it was me, it was me as the object, the thing on the conveyor belt as the mechanics of disease moved me along. I was incidental, not central to what was happening around me. I thought, wrongly, that I was in this alone because I felt that my solo effort to change my own reality was working.

The treatment relies heavily on statistical analyses which describe the past behaviors of populations of patients, and nothing of the future behavior of one person. The treatments frighten so deeply and completely because they are blunt weapons against disease in our culture that washes us in both the real and the mythical claims that medicine can be practiced with precision. We communicate to ourselves the illusions of precision through the ceaseless announcements of technologies. But as most doctors try to explain and describe treatments for cancer, they mention that they did not know what kind of patterns I would face.

"Some get very sick, some don't get sick at all....there is really no predictor about that," the oncologist told me. Then he hastened to add, "but we do know that it works in most cases of carcinoma. "

"How sick will I get?" I asked him.

"I just don't know. A lot will depend on your attitude."

"What does that mean, my attitude? What part of my attitude? What should I do to get ready for it?'

He tried again to tell me what he knew, but he really had no effective way to communicate the idea they simply do not know the connections with in each person in how the character and the spirit receive the treatment. They know how the blood and the biology of the body receives it, but we do not how our minds receive the idea that we are being poisoned to heal. I think in that short interview we each knew we are a great complex mix of mysteries.

I got very sick. The nurse in the oncology ward was a very beautiful and gentle lady whom I never forget, but cannot every recall either her name or face only her character. She would visit with me and tell me that she knew I would grow strong again. She asked me to visit with the younger patients and convince them to get up and walk.

"You will beat this," she said once, just plainly. The only sentence she spoke after watching me a while.

"I don't know how you say that. You know how much this hurts, and you must know what the pain does to people. You must know how this can drive a person crazy, this idea that one bag holds the other in balance, with the sick guy in the middle."

She looked away, embarrassed at my response. "What's the matter?" I asked.

"That's the point, Mark. I see you and others here every day, but I really don't know I see it, but I don't know it. Sometimes I feel like I am nothing more than a spectators."

"But we need spectators... as long as they are also fans," I told her.

Consider how to act toward the sick. The person who is trying to heal uses all means available: intellectual, psychological, physical, emotional, and spiritual aspects. When all connect, the synergistic affect itself is a success, and whether the end physical result is life or death from disease is no longer the issue. So, the essential question for a friend who has cancer is not what or how it happened, but rather, *Now that you have your cancer, what will you do with it?*

I found that recovered patients are largely anonymous. As a society, we expect them to go back into the society and hide. To never again mention the dreaded illness they had. The key word is had. We put the disease in the past, as if it was historical, but we know better. We know the disease does not die. We may kill it, fend it off, but we know it is not eradicated. So we seek out the symbols, the icons of our culture who are afflicted with any experience of disease and we expect them to carry the day for all of us. We want name recognition, rather than studies of who got well. Somehow, we collectively want some social psychology that assures us that diseases are things of the ancient past, and that we need not worry of them any longer. It is an old story. But disease, and especially cancer, is with us always. It can instruct as well as it can frighten and I learned more from cancer than I ever would have imagined before I got it. I think one of the major psychological challenges I had was that when I got cancer the first time, I did precisely what was expect. As I dutifully sought my "old self" I fought it on a physical level, and it took me some time, but I learned first hand it was fare stronger and deep than that. I heard these questions hundreds of times, and they were questions for which I never found answers.

"Is there anything I can do?"

"Just call if you need anything."

"What do you need?"

Unimpressed by such talk, Debra and I both did not know what to ask and never called anyone who talked like that. Instead, we will always remember and appreciate the friends who called and asked the kids favorite dish so that they could cook it and bring it over. We remember the people who just showed up after a call to the kids out for the day. The people who took a grocery list so that she did not have to go. The people who were considerate enough to know that every day you care for your husband in chemotherapy is a day you cannot go to the store or the to the laundry, or name something unless you have help. The family was in crisis, and when in crises, people do not have time or perspective to think about what comes next, they think about the next hour, next morning, the next nap, the next invitation to some party of some weekend.

"THE DON'TS."

- Don't ask, "What do you need?" Instead, offer something. Wash the car, fix the car. Do the windows, clear out the garage, do the shopping. Do something.

- Don't use the patient, your friend, as a way to learn about the particular disease. If you want to learn, go to a library, bookstore or a medical class.

- Don't use "sound bites," the television and radio social psychology that bombards us. For the patient who has entered chemotherapy, cancer is much more complex than the feature on some new drug, new surgical technique, or diet plan that is usually featured. His problems are not easily solvable with some 'silver bullet' philosophy. The only way to understand what happened is to learn to understand what continues to work on the body; it is a matter of chemical and biological relationships, including those that interact with the medicine. There is really no other experience to compare with it, unless the patient himself or herself choose to compare one.

- Don't ask, "What kind of cancer do you have? (or did you have?"). The first question can prompt an involved answer, and if you are prepared to invest some time to listen, then don't ask. Also, think for a moment that if the patient has not told you to begin with what kind it is then they probably do not want to discuss it. Instead, allow the patient to tell the story as they want. Try to understand that much of this can be very private in nature and question itself can be intrusive. Let them be, on this score and just listen to what they want to tell you.

- Don't use words and codes you do not understand: Using the same thinking as in the case above, try not to ask about "remission," which has specific clinical and personal meaning to a patient, unless you know the case and the person. As a cancer patient, I have learned that many of the "code words" of cancer are widely misused, and "remission" is among the most commonly used and least understood. The words excite certain hope, fear, emotion, and elation. This is all fair if the well meaning visitors understand that they are sending messages with these words that may be quite powerful and excite e powerful reactions in their friend.

- Don't ignore the patient, your friend, your loved one, to visit
  with others. Instead, visit and socialize with them by
  including the person who you presumably came to see.

- Don't compare one case to another, especially in terms of
  statistics or survival rates, or anecdotes about t some one you
  once knew.

- Don't talk about them if they are not there, unless it is
  something you would say in their presence.

- Don't use conjecture, as if somehow something in the recent
  past has caused it. Many do this, I have found, in the honest
  effort that if they can somehow help the person to explain it,
  then somehow it will make them more knowledgeable and
  more able to deal with it. For example, in my case, "Do you
  think if you got it again because you went to the Sinai? It
  was very hot there and they say heat can cause a virus which
  can cause a tumor?"

I could not revisit any decision or time of the past, not to
change it anyway. What is done is done. The much more
effective technique, in my opinion, it for the friend to prompt the
patient to look forward, not back, to ask their own assessment o
of what they think of their own future, to set the sights on
something positive.

On one particularly painful evening while I was in
chemotherapy, eight different friends came to my bedside. They
did not arrange a group visit; it just worked out that way. They
were all upbeat and made jokes. They thought I was asleep, and
they began to talk about my surgery. With my eyes still closed, I
told them that if they really wanted to know about the scars, the

two incisions on the sides (from which each testicle was removed) led to the long arrow in the middle, and it makes an arrow, which tells them where to go. As they began to leave, someone said, still laughing, "Well what can we do for you?" My answer was without hesitation,

Paint my house.

They all laughed, telling me my sense of humor had returned, and then they all left, at once. Everyone thought I was kidding, but I was serious. I really wanted someone to paint my house, to check my roof, and to do some other chores that I meant to get on that spring. Admittedly, I was testing them a bit and it was clearly my fault for allowing them all to think it was a joke. I should have told them I meant it. But I wanted to see the reaction to a practical request from a friend who is sick. I think somehow we simply do not believe or do not listen seriously to someone who is seriously sick and weak.

THE "DO'S."

- Do recognize the intellectual and emotional and psychological and spiritual sides to people. Try to answer their needs.

- Do seek out all means to fight the disease. Medical, spiritual, intellectual, emotional, physical. As mentioned earlier, find the facts about the cancer involved. As much as I consider the value of the work of Bernie Siegel, I also came to realize that no matter what the approach toward positive thinking, some cancers advance and kill. So, I think it is very

important for the patient to do personal assessment of the
facts of the disease relative to the life of that patient. I write
this not to criticize any of the great work by doctor Seigel
nor others. I wrote it to say that all means should be used,
and the patient should avoid any over reliance one technique.

• Do show as much as you say you care. Do something
  material. If you do not have time or energy to call or to talk,
  then don't.

• Do find humor.

• Do find a way to show you are in support when they fail,
  when they cannot make it through the day, when the self
  doubt takes over and wins out for a time. Find a way to let
  them know it is OK to fail, but not for too long. Instead of
  listening to the question, "Why me?" ask your friend to
  instead try, "Now that you have the disease, what will you
  do with it?"

• Do examine your own spirituality. Consider what you
  believe happens upon death. Then, if you feel close enough
  to the person, allow them to express this what they feel about
  it. Give signs that it is fine to talk to you in confidence. Do
  not assume that past behavior is a model for how they will
  feel or act now or in the near future. Their outlook on
  spirituality may well be changing, and they may be looking
  for someone with whom to share that. If your friend is in
  need of expressing the spiritual, do not assume he wants you
  to find the chaplain, minister, or rabbi. Let him do it to you.
  Some of the most spiritual people and exceptional

counselors have no connection to religion, at least not in a
professional way.

- Do communicate openly, with consideration toward the
  patient's feelings and the patient's point of view.

Shortly after my recovery, when I finally had all strength
back and my diet and exercise were fairly normal, on one of my
trips to follow up for the doctor, I considered the day. On the
way to the office, I noticed a few other patients going to see him
and they were not very well. I considered what I had done so far
that day that I could not have done only months earlier. It begins
with awakening, then rising. For me, these were usually two
different tasks. It would take the better part of an hour to garner
the strength to rise after I awoke. Consider how routine you take
the ability to rise from bed, go to the bathroom, wash up and take
a shower, and then shave, dress and move on. Now consider
every one of those moves, each physical movement, slowed to
only a third of normal speed. The minutes, then the hours moved
beyond me, and still I was not done in the bathroom while the
pain continued to mount. I took some measure of success
because this morning maybe you can do it without assistance.
But a certain move, maybe while you put on pants or raise the
toothbrush and some residual odor from last night ignites sudden
vomiting takes dashes your brief self-congratulations and you
know you still cannot awaken without assistance. Now walk out
to the kitchen and try to decide what to eat and how to eat it. A
piece of toast? A bit of cereal? Can you stand the odor of bread
in the toaster? It depends on the kind of bread, depends on the
residue in the toaster. You sense all the odors, many too strong to
allow you to stay in the kitchen, so you try to find a place in your
house where there are no scents, and you cannot. The only
constant in this day is the nausea.

As I sensed my own breathing, I saw patterns, both rhythmic and chaotic, within the same breaths. As I negotiated the next waves of illness asked out loud,

> *Is it the lack of sleep, the chemicals, or is it something in my mind?*

The answers of course are not there, and if they were they would not matter to you nearly as much as the effort to ask the question. As in many things that involve human effort, the questions presume the problems. But at least a hundred times a day the small physical action takes away all your meager strength and you seek out the reasons again and again. The reactions within you depend on the moment, and may depend on the microscopic forms of both chemotherapy metals at work and their reactions within the microscopic tunnels of your membranes, cells, and nodes, and hopefully in the small battles between chemical and cancer that rages. But the patterns of such battles are yet to be solidified and codified in your own mind. I struggled, physically and mentally, to help in the effort while sensing that the chaos within me in fact has patterns, but I cannot yet hope to know them.

For Debra, the impact came with the shock of a frozen wind in the night. From nowhere she could expect, the chill that robs not only the breath but now robbed her of the most personal and private of choices for a woman: to have or not have children. The cancer had determined that she could bear no more children. The insinuations and then the outright advice on the private matter from casual acquaintances seemed to be all around her. "You have two kids, count your blessings." "It could have been much worse. It might have spread, he might have died." "I don't see why you are complaining. You have to think of him. He's the

one that got sick, not you." "Why can't she just be happy that he
is OK?"

No manner of code words could account for the reality that
this was now out in the open for anyone who knew us even
causally to comment upon, the fact that I could no longer father
children. There was very little consideration to her point of view
and her feelings. It was an emotional event, one she needed to
work through. This invasive disease delivered her a very
personal and private kind of suffering, one she had not expected.

A fact of life within our culture, I think, is that we fear not
only the sickness, but also the people who are sick. We may
begin the relationship with the sick friend by visits and calls, but
we soon grown weary of it. As a society, we tend to personalize
it too much, and begin to think that the sight of a sick persona is
too hard to take. If you watch carefully in a hospital ward of
seriously ill patients, you will see many signs of how most
visitors are far more concerned with their own mental outlook
and appearances than they are with the patients. Some of that
may be connected to the idea that as a rule; we do not associate a
person's appearance as valid if it is in pain.

One window into how a loved one is handling cancer
treatments is the waiting room in an oncology clinic. Think
about what you see, first in general, then in particular relation to
friend or loved one. You will get an insight into the world of
chemotherapy. Many people will lightly consider the patient and
will say that they did not visit, because they wanted to "give
them time to get better," or "let them have time alone at home
with the family, or some other such aphorism. Those who make
statement s such as these are not to be criticizes, that would be a
bit cruel and without purpose. They are to be understood, I think
in terms of just how terribly hared it is for most of us to face our
own inevitable mortality. So if some wish to distance themselves
from the sick, it is understandable.

The original purpose of this was probably not to cure, but to separate. It was a place where people could go to die so that those who are not sick would somehow feel like they had provided some place where the infections would be apart from the community, and further, someplace where the living were not bothered with the dying. It makes us feel better to think that those not in hospital are not sick. But it has never been true. Much has progressed, and medicine has isolated disease. We are no longer so threatened by the sick. Or do we maintain such a fear? Do we still distance ourselves from the people, as well as from the diseases they carry?

My now anonymous nurse moved lightly and quietly, like a dancer. Her soft but strong eyes looked into me and pierced my fog. The chemicals filtered my vision and my hearing, but I focused well enough to hear her curiosity about the red roses sent by my friend Roger Spiller.

"Why did he send those?" she asked me. I smiled as I thought of Roger, who has studied and taught so much about the human dimensions of history to so much of the officer corps. One of his favorite stories is Stephen Crane's classic, *The Red Badge of Courage.*

"Roses..." I said, "...are his way to tell me that the battle is within me. The main character of the book is named Henry Fleming. He is a young boy who wants to perform, to prove he is a man, as he faces his first battle in the Civil War. But he discovers that in the face of great danger, his world is now different, frightening, overpowering. The first time he faces the enemy, he runs, and in running he is hurt badly and gets bandaged. Then when he has his wound, his "badge," his manhood is proven to others, but his battle within grows more serious. The story is filled with irony..."

I surprised myself at how I recalled some of the details of the story. It occurred to me while I spoke to her that the character was also insignificant in the world, or so it first appeared. I recalled a spot, and took up the small paperback that Roger had sent me. It took me a minute to find the passage ...*he had grown to regard himself merely as a part of a vast blue demonstration. His province was to look out, as far as he could, for his personal comfort...he felt that in this crisis his laws of life were useless. Whatever he had learned of himself was here of no avail...* He was incidental in this world of battle. He was not the central part of anything until he looked within himself. Was I only incidental to this world of cancer and chemotherapy?

"Let them know it hurts," she said quietly.

"What? Let who know what hurts?" I answered.

"Patients, people. Let them know that it hurts to be sick. I think most people do not think about what happens here, in these wards, and doctors write about it all the time, and some patients, but tell people how much work this is and how it can be done, but that they must do it. Most patients are shocked by that, and most never do get it. So many people think cancer will just go away once they have surgery. Sometimes I think your kind of cancer is the hardest, harder mentally than a tumor that everyone knows is life threatening, because then the end is clear, they will either live or die. But in so many cases like yours, the story is more involved. Everyone seems to think it is just a matter of take out the small tumor and then it is over. But it isn't. We talk about you here a lot. Tell your story to people," she said. "Most people do not know at all what to do, how to start, how to feel, and so few realize they have to heal themselves in this. You seem to know that. Tell them about it."

She touched my hand, she smiled and she left. She thanked me, and I thanked her. The room was filled with ideas when we parted, and it was filled with roses. Her image never again crossed my mind until years later. Whoever she is, I thank her.

But I lived for Debra's visits. Her footsteps, smell her perfume, her unmistakable voice each changed my day. The comfort of her was in both the familiar and in the expectation of what would come again later. If my time were divisible into a series of units that fit the patterns of the pain of the chemotherapy, I would have found that there were noticeable patterns in my reactions, and it was the combinations of these patterns that allowed me to cope with effects of the poison, which in turn allowed d me to heal. But it was the search, more than the discovery, that healed me.

When my time was measured by the divisions of the clock, the chemotherapy doses of four hours were invasions that damaged and hurt. I felt that each bag was a hot blast wind while I was exposed and vulnerable, caught out in the open with no protection. I was powerless to stop the extreme effects; it all came upon me at once and there was no pattern that I could find. But later, on consideration, I thought of the treatments more like pools within rivers. There were patterns to them, if I looked at them as smaller pieces, within places in the river. The feelings of the chemotherapy swirled rather than flowed. The pain and the panic were there, true, and if looked upon as a whole, those effects never left. But when I considered it in its pieces, the pain, despite its heat and intensity, was followed briefly by instants of elation at the surety of recovery. There was a sensing that this was for the good, that the temporary effects would pass and this would do its designed purpose. The chemotherapy was not all confusion; there were patterns in its seemingly random nature.

Maybe there are threads; material connections still to be found, yet to be illuminated. For now, though, sciences are not yet able to deliver a piece of random information in science to dissect the tumor. It seems that we still rely on the static, historical statistics, which describe very little relevant information to most individual patients. But in my mind and character, I sensed that the patterns of pain, elation, and depression and fear connected to the particles of cancer and to their reactions to the chemotherapy agents. I sensed, felt, and began to believe in the connections between the physical, spiritual, medical elements that worked at points in time. If I could somehow trick time, freeze it, then there might be new ways to approach the healing. I neither accepted nor reject the orthodox methods of tetrameter, just as I neither accepted nor rejected the so-called mind body philosophies. I worked kept working both my brain and my body and my mind to get well. I desperately tried to take charge of my healing.

I think this is one reason many people are surprised at their own reactions to cancer patients. Perhaps it is because almost instinctively we see ourselves sin every sick person, and maybe there is something genetically that we all carry which tells us we are looking at death. And while we are born with genetic codes that tell us when parts of life will change and eventually end, we teach ourselves that all death is to be avoided, no matter the cost. The natural tension between what we teach ourselves and what we carry within our genes comes crashing into our practical world when we witness people dying of cancer; being slowly and painfully consumed, dying when some vital organ finally fails. One reason for the lack of practical dialogue about what to "do" about cancer is that we still do not know it springs from our behavior and environment, or if it is built in to us from the beginning, and therefore the issue simply becomes too philosophical and too hard to address in a practical way.

I did not rely on the statistics. I questioned them. Truth and statistics do not make a healthy marriage, not even an enjoyable date, as the two dance past our eyes to tunes we sometimes recognize, sometimes not. We tend to mix them up and allow them to color and cloud our thinking as we look for solid points of important truths. The material parts of the dance, unfortunately, remain defined by so many numbers. They have their use, the numbers, but when considering things about medical science and things about healing, the statistics do not mean much to the patient. What matters to the patient is the truth, and all truths are relevant to the assumptions about how we live. The statistics, on the other hand, are not at all about the patient, but the group, the population of patients, and they cannot predict the future outcome of a case.

Each four-hour block of chemotherapy seemed to have its own character of unpredictable moments when sickness would overwhelm and other moments, under seemingly identical conditions, when the chemicals would have an opposite, almost uplifting effect. I noticed patterns to these assaults. They would begin with waves of heat, then pain, then nausea, then overwhelming fatigue. But there was more. There was a pattern to the patterns, as if a picture of the entire graph of my reactions would somehow produce a predicable series of painful events spike on a graph, to be followed by a time that I could not tell what it would be, save that it would be completely different form what it was some minutes earlier. Rather than become upset of this unpredictability, I played with it in my head. It added variety to my day and as I played with it I also explored my visualization methods. This would continue day and night at unpredictable times. At times, I thought it related only to the timing of when they administered the drugs, but I learned a few days that it seemed to bear no relation to the timing of the drug, but rather something within my internal reactions. Each time the pattern was the same, I would go through the sickness and then some time later engage in visualization.

One might conclude that these patterns were directly connected to the alkalyting agents and the series of chemotherapy treatments. But the medicines alone could not explain for me what was beginning within me. Alone in that

room, visions of my future and past mixed together. I came to
think that although the oncologist had dutifully calculate the
chemical equations, he did not know the outcome of what he
planned, not without me. Only I could influence the results, he
would tell me. But I did not know how to do it.

From where was I to take my signals? Surely not from the
population of other patients. The statistics for thinking, for
finding the patterns, not for building some kind of belief, some
kind of theology of medicine. "A thirty per cent chance of
recovery." Does that mean that seven of ten people with this die
in five years? What does that mean to me? Or does it mean
something else? How is the term "free of disease " interpreted in
my case? Does it mean some length of time without treatment?
Does it speak to some quality in a life? Does it mean free of
physical pain? Over what period of time are the statistics valid?
What is the base of the basis of them? All of these questions may
apply. None of them may apply. There are no models by which
to fill in the puzzles of cancer. The patient can find only shades
within shades, and only after they have examined their own
process in life.

What do mortality rates mean? Doctors are not imbued with
the qualities of prophets. They simply relate to patients what
they think the historical "statistics" are about a case "like theirs."
Then the patient works his time. Like clocks in the head and in
the soul, they internally set the time that will start them on a path
to validate that time. It gives them purpose. Their purpose is to
design a strategy for the last months of their life, so they try to
get things in order for the departure. When the tasks are done, so
too are they.

When Debra rescued me a second time from the oncology
ward, I saw small tears in the nurses' eyes. Once again, there
was little of my weight and frame left. The poisons had done
their damage. I walked the hallways all night before e she came

to get me, the IV pole inextricably tied to my vein. I marched for
hours and I cried, not out of fear, but out of realization that I had
made it once again. I was thirty seven years old, had done what I
had to date in my life, and I asked first myself and then God how
I was gong to live this time forward. I moved. Whey did all this
fit together for me to continue, it might have run its course in
such a different way.

When she came to get me, we could have been playing out
one of those poignant scenes in the movie of the wrongly
accused prisoner who awaits his release at the gate, awaiting the
arms of his long parted lover. No matter how much good the
experience was for him, he never longs to go back to it. A friend
helped her fold me into the car and we managed to not talk about
any of until I was completely out of sight of the hospital, as if the
building might hear what I said and pull me back to it.

My senses were all on edge, sharp and active. Smells,
aromas of food, even inflections in people's voices and eye
movements were very new to me. My field of vision seemed to
expand, and from the very beginning I wanted to move and to
use the newfound senses. I walked, then jogged, then ran. I had
to move.

With a newly discovered sense of balance, once again I
joined in this intricate and intimate dance with disease. Every
day began to count, but none too much, as I accepted the changes
within and moved into skills a bit higher than those of the boxer.

8 WHICH WAY?

By now, the New Jersey Turnpike has probably led billions of people to places they did not want to go. It is one of life's necessary, if not most inviting, trails. In October of 1990, it guided us to another new beginning. I did not want to leave the Hudson Valley, New York City, and this departure was far more difficult than any previous trips. But one measure of growth and healing is movement, and it was time for me to move. My schedule required two courses before taking command at Fort Benning, Georgia. One was at Fort Jackson, South Carolina, and one was at Fort Leavenworth, Kansas. It made the time between August and our departure from West Point in November very short. The future, if not the turnpike, held hope.

An infantry training battalion is a great mix of discipline, hard work, and promise. The present and the future meld in the hopes of thousands of young men each year as they work to begin adventures in the Army and the infantry. Too busy to think much about their relatively short pasts, most value their future far more than their past. After only a few days on post, we moved into a home on the third green of the golf course. Fort Benning is an enormous place that seems to gobble up most of Columbus, Georgia as well as the Chattahoochee River and part of Alabama. A few hours after I took command, I went to an

obstacle course with a company that was within three weeks of
their graduation into the Army. As I moved through the course
with them, I realized the fun as well as the importance of what
this was about. These were kids, not much older than Sean
really, and I was their "old man." On my jog along the course, a
soldier panicked at the top of a log some thirty feet in the air. He
froze. I could have helped him, but I decided to leave it to the
drill sergeant.

"You're in charge, sergeant," was all I said. Then I got out of
his way and the company commander and I positioned us at a
spot to carefully observe. I was watching for the relationship
between drill sergeant and scared soldier, and I was also
watching for the relationship between the captain and his
company. The most lasting impression was that drill sergeant,
first sergeant, and captain all knew this soldier, and they knew
all their soldiers. A sense of teamwork is what brought the
frightened trainee back to the ground, and when he went back up
to complete his task, he had the backing of his peers and his
leadership. It was a good way to begin.

If one wanted to compare the cadets I left at West Point to
the soldiers entrusted to me at Fort Benning, the only way to find
a measure of difference would be in opportunity. The talent, the
aptitude for learning, the patriotism, and the sense of self-
development between average cadet and average soldier was
very comparable. In many cases, the distinction between West
Point cadet and soldier in training is little more than opportunity
and rate of growth. It is not in intellect or in physical aptitude.

Throwing myself into the job, I did physical training every
day beginning at about five thirty each morning. By midday I
would have been with at least one, maybe two of the five
companies. The training cycles went six days a week for
fourteen weeks. Saturdays were training days. Within a few
weeks I had a very good sense of what needed work. I enjoyed

all of it. It was not only "good therapy," it was genuinely
important work for me. True, the conditions of the impending
war demanded extra effort at every job in the Army, and not only
because I knew it was last chance I would get to command again.
Each of these reasons was valid enough. But there was an even
more important reason for me to give myself to the battalion; it
was about the future.

The battalion was filled with up to a thousand trainees at a
time, under the leadership and tutelage of one hundred and
twenty officers and non-commissioned officers, and our job was
to build then into the best soldiers we could, war or peace,
politics and policy notwithstanding. I was there a few weeks
when someone approached me with a surprise question.

"We were a little concerned about your physical condition."

"What were you concerned about?"

"Oh no, don't get me wrong. Now that we have seen you, we
know you're all right. Hell, I mean anyone who has seen you at
PT (physical training) knows you are healthy."

I was beginning to fail another test of my self-control. "You
know I 'm fine, you say, and how do you know that?" I had to
decide very quickly whether to challenge him or to let it pass. I
danced with each option for a while.

"Well, you know, what happened to you and all."

"And just what is it that you think happened?"

"Well, someone said you had cancer. We heard about your
treatments and I just wanted to be sure you were OK. That's all."

I was learning to live with men's thinly veiled curiosities about
my testicles.

My first talk to the cadre of the battalion began by stating
that I wanted them to hear about what I valued from me
personally, and I wanted to offer all of them a condensed version
of what was now a long story about me. I told them that I had
recovered from cancer and that both of my testicles had been

removed. With the hundred or so officers and non-commissioned officers in the room, you could have heard a pin drop. I told them about how I looked upon them, how I valued what they did and who they were, and that we would work together, communicate openly, take care of each other and our families, and train the soldiers. Then I went on to describe the story about cancer. We began to connect.

I ended my first talk to the 4th Battalion, 36th Infantry by telling them they were not just a collection of individuals, but they were a battalion. And tighter we would together we would build a "Family Support Group," something normally associated with units in the Army that deployed to a theater of war. Then I told them I would see them at physical training in the early morning and at some training site throughout the day. Desert Shield loomed over the Army and the country as each week and then each month led into what would clearly be a shooting war. We did our part and a little more as we did what was necessary to meet the demands of the Army. I told them this was the art of the possible, and that they were the artists.

On the day I took command of the battalion, the news featured a story that said that the Chairman of the Joint Chiefs of Staff, General Powell, and the Secretary of Defense, Richard Cheney, visited General Schwarzkopf in Saudi Arabia and agreed to support the operation with the addition of the Army's Seventh Corps stationed in Europe. It would amount to an increase of about one hundred thousand more soldiers to the desert. All talk of solving this by some "non military" means and the troops "being home by Christmas" had ended, and it seemed that the only uncertainty was about when the shooting would begin. Then came a presidential order to recall mobilized soldiers. Under certain provisions of law, the President may recall service people who are still in what is known as the "Individual Ready Reserve," or "IRR," a status kept for six years after one leaves the active force. The soldiers the Army called began with groups of volunteers, beginning in August, for specified jobs, the biggest being truck drivers. But as time went on the Army found it needed to get many more, and we moved beyond volunteers.

Many received telegrams to go to Fort Benning in about ten days to report to for retraining and active duty. Most were married, many were in college. Many were quite happy to come back, some were not. The majority were in their mid to late twenties. As the mobilization developed, we received them, processed them back into service, trained them, and then shipped them on to designated places around the Army. Most were to take the place of other soldiers who had been moved away from their jobs to the assignments in Saudi Arabia. It was building into a scenario of large proportion. This was not very different from other wars in our past, except that this was the first war in which we mobilized an all-volunteer force.

Each soldier had a story. Until the telegrams arrived, most had never considered how they would return to the Army. Late one night, a lady sought me out to tell me something I have never forgotten.

"I just want you to know that my son was a soldier once, and he is now in college with a young wife and a child. He fought in Panama He won't complain about coming back, but why does my son have to go again when so many never go at all?"

The mother's question has an almost haunting quality. In any society with voluntary military service, there is an old issue: the tension between freedom and obligation. While political decisions and policies pursue policies that involve normal or routine tasks for the country's military, there are the routine questions of recruitment, officer recruitment, careers, entitlements, and budgets, among others. But when any policy approaches the means of war, then we change.

The changes may be dramatic, or it may be slight and subtle, and take place over some time. But as a society and a military, we change. Though the changes may be small, they matter a great deal because they reflect what we value as we commit people to war. All of that is normally understood by the volunteer and professional force. But the question of our values, there hanging between the mother and me at Sand Hill on a midnight in January 1990, was not about our professional volunteers, it was in fact about her son, once a volunteer soldier, who had now been recalled. Will my son have to fight in another war?

It is never easy to be an infantryman. Marches, runs, physical training, and hundreds of newly learned skills that are trained to some level of standard of performance. The cadre, the drill sergeants, first sergeants, and the officers, were part of an organization highly efficient for its designed purposes. But it needed something a little more. We in the training base during the war worked to build programs and meet requirements in the field at the very dramatic time when the Army was clearly going to war. They had been pulled from their lives, and now we had to prepare them.

My personal drama of cancer was being out paced and overshadowed, even for me, every day by the collective drama of the building for Desert Shield and the looming war. Many of these soldiers who came into the Army expected opportunities and now would graduate from training in a few weeks and possibly go off to war. And wars are usually particularly harsh on two classes of people, civilians, and infantrymen. There is a quiet, almost secret, society that imposes on itself a set of rules that say once we recover, we must go back to be what we were. It imposes on us the notion that whatever the illness or the experience was, it must now be forgotten, largely because the people around us do not want to know about it until it affects them personally. I have found this is an unfortunate but a powerful force. It is unfortunate because many patients feel compelled to try to come away from that notion and what they really require is a modification of that. They need the disease precisely not for what it does to their body, but rather for what it makes them see with their minds and their soul. They needed something to transform their lives, their thinking, and their feelings. But under the enormous pressure of society, they must pretend that all of that is in their past.

As November passed, it became clear that something dramatic was going to happen. One of the first steps was the considerations of mobilization in all its forms and stages. Every Christmas season throughout the Army's training base the entire centers shut down and the soldiers go home for two weeks. In December, the Army leadership decided that the training centers would not take off the normal two weeks in the Christmas season. It was a message, correct and true: in my opinion, that while soldiers were in Saudi Arabia awaiting word for combat, to shut down the training posts for vacation was the wrong message to the rest of the Army. So we trained.

The perspective on this depended largely on who you were and where you were. In the minds of the trainees, it was the most dramatic of moves. Not because they would miss going home, but also because it meant that something very powerful was about to happen to them. And that they were about to be a part of something larger than themselves. The promise of Christmas leave mattered, but not nearly as much as the signal the Army sent with its cancellation.

There were frequent foot marches at night. I liked to talk with the trainees and I liked to listen to what mattered to them. We walked a lot at night. On a night in December, just after we had learned there would be no leave, I was walking on a road march that began in the early afternoon and would stretch long

into the night on its twenty mile course. This company was about
to graduate in a week.

"What do you think about the war, sir? Do you think we will
go to it? They told me that they will probably change my orders.
Probably go to the first division at Fort Riley instead of to
Hawaii. No leave."

"What do you think of that?"

"It's OK with me to go, I just hope we learned the right
things here. What do you think about it sir?"

"What I think does not matter as much as what you do and
think," I answered him. "Keep working, learning, Stay fit, stay
healthy, take care of your buddies, and stay in touch with your
family. You have some great leaders out there in the Army.
Listen to them, help them. Be a good soldier and you'll be fine."

And then I marched up ahead to still another trainee, another
one who might go off to war while we stayed at Fort Benning
and trained. Soldiers know themselves in training, and I would
routinely ask the soldiers a simple question, "What challenges
you the most here?" Most would respond that it was the long
road marches under heavy packs, especially done at night. I
walked on all of these that I could, usually two a week. It was
one way I had to talk with them and to sense how our leadership
cared for them. Most young men simply never thought about
what it takes to walk twenty miles, and their spirits and faces on
completing such rigorous training is a rare thing of beauty and a
testimony to the human spirit.

Graduation from Infantry One Station Unit Training (OSUT)
is not unlike graduation from West Point. Hats do not fly in the
air and it is not done in a football stadium, but parents and wives
and girlfriends come from all over the country and populate the
motels of Columbus, Georgia to see their sons complete a
milestone in their lives. We give them certificates, awards, and
speeches, and tell the parents how much we appreciate the

trusting of the children to the US Army. The scene happens at every training center every Friday morning and it remains one of the enduring strengths of our military. Each soldier has a story: a past and a future, and for a short while some of us are privileged to be a part of their links between the two, their time in training.

In quiet and personal ways, I began to view emotions and behaviors of people through the lens of cancer. Time and distance enabled me to visualize people not only in the present, but images of what they might be in the future. The art of leading people blended with my views on what I had learned about my weaknesses as well as my strengths over the past years' negotiations with cancer. Cancer is after all, about failure, the failure of the immune system to stop some growth or infection or invasion, and life is much more about failure than it is about success. The human side of leading and training, the connections between soldiers' confidence and performance were taking on very personal and practical forms.

A year had passed at Fort Benning when a new and very personal war began for me. I was forced to face a side of the deceitful cancer when it was at its best in deceit and camouflage. It snuck up on me in a way I never would have expected and in a way for which I never could have prepared. Our brigade had nine battalions, and the deputy brigade commander made for ten lieutenant colonels, a rather large organization. Our deputy commander, a man a bit older than most of us, was diagnosed with cancer. He was in his late forties, very healthy, and, by all appearances, everything in his life was in order.

He knew soldiers and knew training, and knew a lot about the infantry.

A very tough guy who was also the perfect gentleman and very gracious, everyone seemed to like him. He was an infantryman who worked his way up through the ranks and in his final years in the Army was first in command of the school system in which officers were trained, and then he came to be our deputy commander at the training center. When he went into the hospital, I did not know how to act.

The cancer was advancing rapidly and the doctors could not operate. It had become too involved with some vital organs. Talk at our conference room table before the start of our staff meetings was always to be the same: we seemed always to recognize his existence, but not his reality.

"Did you see him today?" Some one would start off.

"Yeah, I saw him. He looks good. Getting better. "

"He looks like he might beat it. He seems OK."

And then the routine meeting would begin and no one would say any more of him.

No one ever suggested that he was dying and that we as a group should address that fact. None of us talked about what he and his family might need as he lay dying. Instead, we were fooled by the camouflage. We collectively set the cancer aside. I did not know how to communicate my conflict; I was sympathetic but afraid. I felt I had something to offer to help him, but I also felt I had no right to do so. After all, I did not suffer from cancer and I had recovered. Who was I to tell him how to handle this? I did not know how to approach him.

To those around me, it seemed that my history of two bouts with cancer was completely forgotten. I found people explaining parts of chemotherapy to me in simplistic terms as if I had never heard of it, and they knew these things because they had just visited with him. I came to learn that it is very rare for people to separate their thoughts of suffering from their thoughts of recovery and disease. It may be that some diseases, such as cancer are a bit "too close to home."

At the time, I elected to remain anonymous. I made little effort to remind others what the chemotherapy did to him. My involvement with him became private. I would visit with him regularly, sometimes coming late at night after a day of work, cleaning up just enough before stopping in. We would talk about my day. One day he told me that he did not think he could take the pain any longer. He began to talk of his life and his sons. He was reflective, and hopeful. His talk moved relentless toward his past.

"I could have been a better father. But I guess that is just the way it goes. I wonder where he went."

"Where who went?"

"My son. I told you I had a son, didn't I? Maybe not. I hope he is all right. But I just don't know. He was a hard boy to live with. Then he grew up and left."

"Sometimes that just happens. We don't like to tell ourselves that, but it's true. Sometimes things just happen between people, between fathers and sons, and no one is at fault."

"Like my cancer you mean? You know, I thought I could beat this, I did. But I did not come in on time; I tried to ignore it. And it just got worse. And now look at me. I never told them about my father's cancer. He had the same kind, but I never told the doctors..." He trailed off, then came back with,

"....I think maybe I can beat this. Maybe I will feel better tomorrow."

"Why don't you try eating something?"

"Yes I'll try to eat. Thanks for listening."

About a month later he stopped speaking in the future tense. Though so few seemed to know him personally, everyone came to the ceremonies for him, and everyone had good things to say. But I sensed that we were each there more for our children and ourselves than we were for Ben, and maybe that is part of what this book is about. Maybe. As my friend Marc told me at my father's death, "...funerals are for the living."

Ben left more behind than he could have known.

I also left something behind at Fort Benning. There was the privilege of leading those thousands of young men and the hundreds of cadre members. There was, as always, the satisfaction of the job. But I left something else behind as well. I left some of the cancer there. I began to believe I was "free of disease," and more than in a clinical sense. The cancer had evolved and I had evolved, to a place where the cancer was useful. My cancer was not gone. Rather, it had grown into a valuable tool for my mind and my heart. As we left Fort Benning for yet another move to Carlisle Barracks, Pennsylvania, and then eventually to Yongsan Garrison, Seoul, Korea, my understanding of cancer and recovery grew. I realized what I was leaving behind at Fort Benning. I left the fear.

9 FLOWS AND STEPS

My experiences with cancer have changed me. When I decided to do something with my disease, I faced challenges that I could not anticipate. My story is much more common than it is heroic, much more human than superhuman. Maybe my story can help explain what happens when people recover. The cancer changed my body, and it transformed my self-image. While I have touched that rare intersection of mind, body, and spirit, the picture of health in all areas still eludes.

Men fear this disease. The fear does not spring from some immature fixation on body parts, nor from what may be mistaken as another sort of adolescent attitude, but rather it comes from something of substance. Cancer in general and testicular cancer in particular scares us because it touches what we leave behind. I think that although most men appear to not be interested in it in public, in private they are very willing to investigate. Cancer can make a patient feel robbed of identity because the process and the treatments are clearly clinical and calculated, almost irrespective of the person's character. Growing within our cells, we never know its source. Go a step further and place the invasion in the testicles or other reproductive organs, and the and a kind of border may have passed, beyond which we can no longer clearly know the ways within and around the disease. I think that is why so many appear to not want to discuss it, to simple leave it alone.

The ability to have children, a very personal and private affair, was also a piece of the puzzle of cancer. When I was diagnosed, the last thing that would have occurred to me was the need to visit a sperm bank. When the second case developed, it was too late. The only precaution I took was to protect the remaining testicle during the prophylactic radiation treatments. The shock of the diagnosis completely erased any thoughts of plans for more children. I think it is one matter to decide to no longer have children; I think it is quite another to find that the ability has been stolen. I tried for a while to simply forget it all, but I could not just tuck it away somewhere. The testicles are not central to my story, but neither were they peripheral. Losing the second one carried physiological and psychological messages.

The effects of full testosterone replacement influenced my outlook. I had to learn to control emotions in the face of chemical balances and levels that clearly drove me to emotional highs and lows. How much of that has been "chemical," and how much a part of my new outlook might have made for a valid medical or psychological study, but the most important part to me was that no matter the source of my emotional trials, they were a part of my routine now and I needed to address them.

I did not seek any spiritual or emotional connections with my experiences until much later. For much of my story, I thought I was in this adventure alone. In time, I was able to comprehend why I approached the struggle from behind the protective shroud of that self created image: strong and solitary. The image, though, was not an end but rather it was a transition state to allow me to reenter life with new ways of thinking, to allow me to see the need to change.

I have told much of the physical pain. There have been times since the surgery when I believed that I could recall and re-live the operation. So vivid were these images that I often hallucinated around them. I have recalled the spoken words between surgeons, some familiar, some technical. I can recall the tone of voice, the surprise at the lack of bleeding, the cuts of the knife into the various nodes. Some cuts were accompanied by sharp pain, some by no pain at all. Does the mind have the ability to bring back vignettes, or even to recall all of what happens to us? If so, what might that hold for the art of healing and recovery? The question for me, it seems, is not in how to put the pain and the surgery out of my mind, but rather how to gather the remnants of the experiences and weave them into some fabric that may aid me in the future.

When I first recovered from radiation treatment, and then two years later from chemotherapy, my senses seemed to expand. Where a normal field of vision might be thirty degrees, I had the image that mine was about sixty. I felt I could sense every scent, hear every voice and noise. I felt as though my mind filtered out very little. Everything found a way in because I had not faced the possibility of losing it all forever. I do not propose to estimate how the practice of medicine might limit human suffering. A classic and endless debate that elicits good thoughts, all technically possible, but probably a debate that drives us more toward incorrect conclusions. I do not think the purpose of medicine is to eliminate all suffering. Maybe it is to alleviate physical pain and to enable people to heal themselves and grow. One way to grow is to recognize the value of the physical suffering that is in fact a part of life. Not to embrace it or to welcome it, but to use its for its value and purpose.

What is the value of suffering? An eternal question, maybe, but one worth examination as patients face terribly lonely and stressful scenarios in pain and in culturally driven norms of anonymity. So powerful is our set of expectations that success means complete recovery that most recover from some serious

condition, try to hide it. Not only is it troublesome to share your
post cancerous condition for personal reasons, but it continues to
carry legal and prejudicial baggage as well. If you think not, call
an insurance agent and ask about a policy after being free of
disease for two years.

On one level, the recovered cancer patient is still seen as a
risk. On another level, he or she is a constant remind that cancer
exits within all of us, maybe too painful a reminder. So we
choose to label them anonymous, trying to think of them as once
again "one of us." And this notion of course is very appealing to
most cancer patients, and they cooperate. As much as the Army
helped me to recover, the Army is a very young and healthy
society, and as a rule, we do not discuss who is sick, at least not
for long. When people are very sick they usually leave the Army.
Therefore, my voyage back to both recovery and career within
the Army was a fascinating trip.

In the sport of rock climbing, it is not the length of the route
or the height of the pitch that determines difficulty. Some of the
most difficult challenges can happen only ten feet above the
relative safety of the ground. "Exposure" is a term used to
describe the condition when a climber finds a route that departs
the relative psychological security of some walls around the
route, and the body of the climber hangs out over a lot of air. The
physical parts of the move may not be difficult, but the element
of exposure adds measurable to the difficulty rating. The
psychological element of the climb is a recognized factor in how
to rate a climb. The face of a rock frequently camouflages its
true nature, its difficulty. At first it appears without pattern,
absent any genetic code that might hold clues about how to find
the path. But then with some examination and study, it reveals
itself. It shows the flows within the rock. I think there is such a
thing as "flow" to a rock.

A rock may not be solid. It comes from molten flows. It comes from liquid. Its climb its face, its textures, its patterns, its face. I have met people who train blindfolded so that they can learn to make the moves without the trickery that vision provides, for many times vision obscures the feel and the flow of the route. They practice this so that they may learn their own sense of balance, without regard to the particular rock face. Crazy as it may seem, those who know the sport realize it is a puzzle, and the solutions are mostly internal to the climber. There is a "flow" to a rock, something an experienced climber can sense as the connection to human movement takes hold. I believe the best climbers sense the rock more than they conquer it. They somehow sense the particles within what once made up the molten flow of the rock form, and they connect to them within as part of the particles that make up the human body. I think mountain climbers do not so much conquer peaks as they do join the flow of the natural drift of the particles that make up the ridges and crests. Mountains, with the particles that are they, connect in to the particles of people. To climb, one must first let go of something. It is one of the paradoxes of the sport that to move to secure places, first you must let go, at least for an instant, risk the next move. In hanging on to the security and the apparent frozen position of the held position, there is no relaxation. Instead, there is terribly hard movement in the hands and the feet's muscles in order to maintain the required stillness and stability needed to maintain motionless on a small ledge. Before you can find security in life, first you must let go of some other part of life. You must first do things that will not let you move at all but will freeze you.

The disease stops us cold. It makes us look at who we are, if only for a short time. After the initial look, cases can become amazingly complex or surprisingly simple. In the end, the patient will decide how the disease affects the patient. Even if heroic and monumental struggles result in death, they are not defeated in the world of cancer. A master of camouflage, cancer fools us. We mistake it for something it is not. The mind either works to help the body heal or it checks out and does not work at all. People with far strength far greater than mine have died heroically from cancer, going with dignity, honor and great skill at the game. Those people inspire and instruct as they die. Many people who do not struggle at all and who develop no clear concept of what happened to them live.

I think that men who are afflicted with testicular cancer, whatever their age, should learn about comprehensive cancer care, should consider the use of a sperm bank, and should consult exercise and sports physiologists as well as use all of the orthodox and routine cancer care systems they can find. There is much more to this apparently "curable" cancer than we generally lead ourselves to believe, proving once again, quite possibly, that our complexities may be the source of our healing as well as the source of our illnesses. I do not know how much of this was in my genes, my mind, or my cells. I know that wherever it began, it wove its way into all parts of my life. This should neither surprise nor frighten the relatively young men who contract testicular cancer. It should serve to instruct them to get involved with it from the beginning, to overlook nothing, and to be an active part of the healing. Testicular cancer in my case touched many people who were a part of my life, even some of those whom I had not yet met. I think that is one of the secrets of the disease. It touches so many, yet the one who holds it is privileged to share it or to hide it or to use it in some way. I think cancer will remain connected to our views of mortality. One outcome for me has been a serious self-examination of physical and emotional and spiritual health.

I do not think doctors heal people. I think they set conditions so that people may be allowed to heal themselves. I often tell people, that despite my very high level of personal fitness when all this began, all the miles and the drills lasted about 36 hours once the chemotherapy began. There was little left of me. What was left was the will to recover.

When I got sick the first time, I dealt with cancer in direct and physical ways, ways I knew, ways that others who looked at me could understand. I sensed at first, then I knew with certainty two years later, that the straightforward way did not fit me. And there is the essence. The way in which a person deals with the cancer must fit the person much more than it must fit the cancer. It camouflages well. It is a disease that has transformed the cells of the body, and therefore transformed the body itself. The transformation of a person is not an easy thing, nor is it always positive. But under some circumstances, and I think recovery from cancer is one of those, it is necessary.

It may be in the precise tools that we find hope, idea that if we are willing to negotiate this disease of cells gone crazy that the help lies where it is most unexpected, in the thinking. The idea that I could actively engage my brain, my mind, as well as my spirit and my physical aspects, is what helped me a great deal. That may be why so many doctors and experts who in fact study many patients speak of such abstractions as patients' "relationship" with the disease.

I told my story to offer some hope, to show that I did get better, better than before, form the cancer. I also told it to thank those who knew me, who inspired me, who gave me strength, who prayed for me. I do not know why I got cancer, nor do I especially care. I care about what I did with it. I have felt the rare intersection of the connection between mind, body, and spirit. Never holding to it for very long at one time, the connection is nonetheless now familiar and recognizable.

I do not know the answers to cancer or to testicular cancer, but I do know a few more of the questions. And maybe that is the point of the book. I do not know what cancer is. I know some things that it is not. It is not a static thing, like an infection or a bad tooth, to be removed and then forgotten. It is not a state that some good thinking and emotional support can cure. It is not a dietary condition that some checklist of the top ten healthiest foods can cure. It is not will power alone. But cancer is very complex, and it will always demand intellectual, emotional, physical, and spiritual connections. Involved strategies not only direct and feel good tactics. Surviving it does not mean success; dying of it does not mean failure. Those are measures how we live, not measure of the results of a disease.

I considered my relationship with disease in flows of time past present and future. To do that, I had to re create what it was to me. I began this story with a scene from climbing because the sensations of my numb fingers frightened me. But the same sensations gave me clues about the threads that run through the facets of my lives. The peaks of cancer treatment are not Everest or Rainier, but heights that belong to millions of people in hospital rooms, waiting rooms, and bedrooms. The challenges are in the search for courage required to simply take in the full view of the image in the mirror. I think the greatest of pain happens in the quietest of times, in the loneliest corners of our minds.

Since the cancer, on a few different rock faces and on a few different peaks, I have said prayers for my father, for Wes, and for my sons. I do not know the climbs that await them. Peaks remain all around us; some will hold adventure and wonder. To climb, you first must let something go. Yielding the security of your present position and present hold on life, you risk some safety in the next move, and in the reach for a new place, there is a new puzzle. Reach for something to hold, but not too tightly. I first questioned, then trusted my ability to touch cancer again, if only for moments at a time, steps at a time, while on a climb back.

BIBLIOGRAPHY

Anderson, Kenneth N. and Lois E., editors. *Mosby's Pocket
Dictionary of Medicine, Nursing, and Allied Health.* St.
Louis: Mosby Yearbook, Inc., 1994.

Brunner, Lillian Sholtis, and Suddarth, Doris Smith, Textbook *of
Medical-Surgical Nursing.* Philadelphia: J. B.
Lipponcott Company, 1988.

Burns, Ken, and Ward, Geoffrey, *Baseball.* New York: Alfred A.
Knopf, 1994.

Crane, Stephen, *Red Badge of Courage.* New York Penguin
Books, 1985.

Foucault, Michelle, *Discipline and Punish.* New York: Random
House, 1979.

Frankl, Viktor, *Man's Search for Meaning.* New York
Washington Square Press, 1984.

Gleick, James, *Chaos.* New York: Penguin Books, 1987.

Gruner, Elliott, *Prisoners of Culture.* New Brunswick, New
Jersey: Rutgers University Press, 1993.

Kuhn, Thomas, *The History of Scientific Revolutions.*
Molenar, Dee, *The Challenge of Rainier.* Seattle: The
Mountaineers, 1987.

Siegel, Bernie, *Love, Medicine, and Miracles*. New York: Harper
     and Row, 1990.

Swonger, Alvin K. and Matejski, Myrtle P., Nursing
     Pharmacology.

Tortora, Gerard J. and Grabowski, Sandra Reynolds, *Principles
     of Anatomy and Physiology*, Seventh Edition. New
     York: HarperCollins College Publishers, 1992.

Will, George, *Men at Work*. New York: Harper Collins
     Publishers, 1990.